AF364242

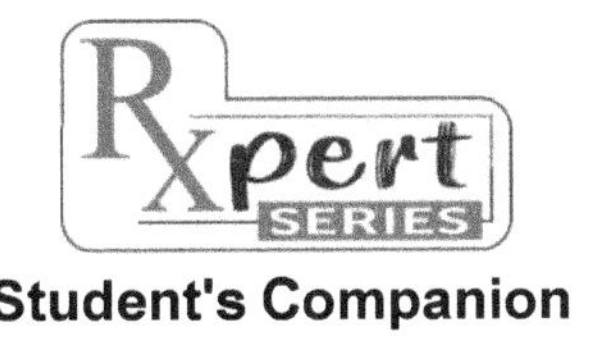

Student's Companion

Quality Assurance

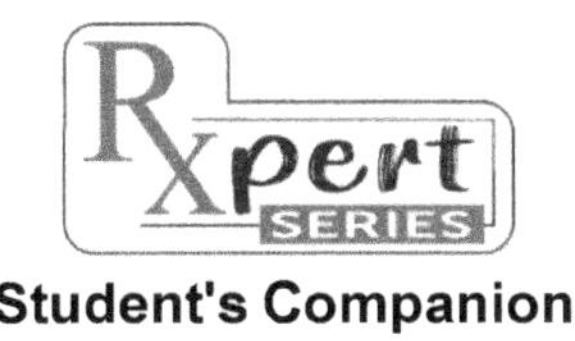

Student's Companion

Quality Assurance

Ankita Dadwal

Associate Professor, Department of pharmaceutics
ISF college of pharmacy, Moga, India

Bhupinder Kumar

Assistant Professor, Department of Pharmaceutical Sciences
HNB Garhwal University, Garhwal, Uttarakhand, India

Raj Kumar Narang

Professor, Department of pharmaceutics
ISF college of pharmacy, Moga, India

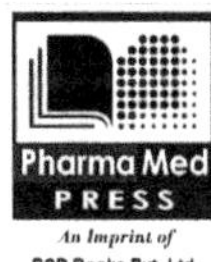

PharmaMed Press

An imprint of BSP Books Pvt. Ltd

4-4-309/316, Giriraj Lane,
Sultan Bazar, Hyderabad - 500 095.

Quality Assurance

by **Ankita Dadwal, Bhupinder Kumar and Raj Kumar Narang**

© 2024, *by Publisher*

Disclaimer: The authors and the publishers have taken due care to provide the authentic, reliable and up to date information related to the subject. However, neither the authors nor the publisher shall be responsible for any liability for any damage caused as a result of use of this book. The respective user must check the accuracy from other sources too.

Published by:

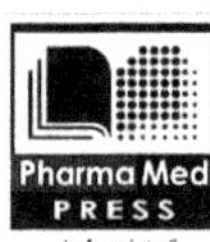

PharmaMed Press

An imprint of BSP Books Pvt. Ltd.

4-4-309/316, Giriraj Lane, Sultan Bazar, Hyderabad - 500 095.
Phone: 040-23445688; Fax: 91+40-23445611
e-mail: info@pharmamedpress.com
www.pharmamedpress.com/pharmamedpress.net

ISBN: 978-93-95039-56-7 (Hardback)

Preface

This book deals with the various aspects of quality control and quality assurance aspects of pharmaceutical industries. It deals with the important aspects like cGMP, QC tests, documentation, quality certifications and regulatory affairs.

The main objectives of this book is that upon completion of the course student shall be able to understand the cGMP aspects in a pharmaceutical industry, Appreciate the importance of documentation, understand the scope of quality certifications applicable to pharmaceutical industries, understand the responsibilities of QA & QC departments.

This book is the outcome of our personal teaching and research expertise in the field of pharmacy. We are optimistic and certain that it will be examined and modified frequently to enhance students' learning experiences. We are also appreciative of the cooperation, support, and advice from our publishers' editorial board.

We anticipate that both teachers and students will find this guidebook to be of great value.

-Authors

Contents

Chapter – 2

Industrial Organization, Personnel, Equipment and Raw Materials

Chapter – 3

Quality Control

Chapter – 4

Complaint

Chapter – 5

Calibration and Validation

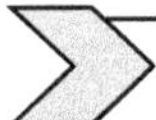 **UNIT 1**

Quality Assurance and Quality Management Concepts

1.1   Introduction

Quality is an important factor when it comes to any product or service. With the high market competition, quality has become the market differentiator for almost all products and services. Therefore, all manufacturers and service providers out there constantly look for enhancing their product or the service quality.

In order to maintain or enhance the quality of the offerings, manufacturers use two techniques, quality control and quality assurance. These two practices make sure that the end product or the service meets the quality requirements and standards defined for the product or the service.

There are many methods followed by organizations to achieve and maintain required level of quality. Some organizations believe in the concepts of Total Quality Management (TQM) and some others believe in internal and external standards.

The standards usually define the processes and procedures for organizational activities and assist to maintain the quality in every aspect of organizational functioning. When it comes to standards for quality, there are many. ISO (International Standards Organization) is one of the prominent bodies for defining quality standards for different industries. Therefore, many organizations try to adhere to the quality requirements of ISO. In addition to that, there are many other standards that are specific to various industries. As an example, SEI-CMMi is one such standard followed in the field of software development.

Since standards have become a symbol for products and service quality, the customers are now keen on buying their product or the service from a certified manufacturer or a service provider. Therefore, complying with standards such as ISO has become a necessity when it comes to attracting the customers.

1.1.1 Quality Control

Many people get confused between quality control (QC) and quality assurance (QA). Let's take a look at quality control function in high-level. As we have already discussed, organizations can define their own internal quality standards, processes and procedures; the organization will develop these over time and then relevant stakeholders will be required to adhere by them.

The process of making sure that the stakeholders are adhered to the defined standards and procedures is called quality control. In quality control, a verification process takes place. Certain activities and products are verified against a defined set of rules or standards.

Every organization that practices QC needs to have a Quality Manual. The quality manual outlines the quality focus and the objectives in the organization. The quality manual gives the quality guidance to different departments and functions. Therefore, everyone in the organization needs to be aware of his or her responsibilities mentioned in the quality manual.

1.1.2 Quality Assurance

Quality Assurance is a broad practice used for assuring the quality of products or services. There are many differences between quality control and quality assurance. In quality assurance, a constant effort is made to enhance the quality practices in the organization. Therefore, continuous improvements are expected in quality functions in the company. For this, there is a dedicated quality assurance team commissioned.

Sometimes, in larger organizations, a 'Process' team is also allocated for enhancing the processes and procedures in addition to the quality assurance team. Quality assurance team of the organization has many responsibilities. First and foremost, responsibility is to define a process for achieving and improving quality.

Some organizations come up with their own process and others adopt a standard process such as ISO or CMMi. Processes such as CMMi allow the organizations to define their own internal processes and adhere by them.

Quality assurance function of an organization uses a number of tools for enhancing the quality practices. These tools vary from simple techniques to sophisticated software systems. The quality assurance professionals also should go through formal industrial trainings and get them certified. This is especially applicable for quality assurance functions in software development houses.

Since quality is a relative term, there is plenty of opportunity to enhance the quality of products and services. The quality assurance teams of organizations constantly work to enhance the existing quality of products and services by optimizing the existing production processes and introducing new processes.

1.1.3 GMP (Good Manufacturing Practices) and Requirements of Premises, Plant and Equipment

In order to ensure production of quality drug formulation, it is necessary on the part of the manufacturer to follow well established and ethical approach involving different operations of manufacture. It was on several occasions discussed in professional meetings and conferences that there is a need for well set mandatary guidelines required to be followed by manufactures of different dosage formulations. It was with this background; Good Manufacturing Practices under Schedule M were made mandatory conditions for manufacturing operations of pharmaceutical formulations.

The quality of drug formulations is the sole responsibility of the manufacturer. He has to ensure the production of desired quality formulations and their stability until, the formulation reaches the consumer across the retailing counter. The Schedule M is covered under Rules 71, 74, 76 and 78 and is in two parts.

Part I deals with GMP relating to factory premises and materials.

Part II deals with requirement of plant and equipment.

1.1.4 PART I: Factory Premises and Materials (Salient Features)

- **General Requirements**

  Good location; free from contamination due to sewage, drain, fumes, dust, smoke, etc.; hygienic conditions; prevention of entry of insect and/or rodents; interior surface of premises should be smooth; adequate lighting; proper ventilation; humidity control; underground drainage; concealed electrical and sanitary fittings in the premises; supply of pure water; regular cleaning and disinfection of premises; proper treatment of waste water; pollution control and disposal of pollutants.

- **Warehousing Area**

  Adequate area for orderly warehousing of various categories of materials; adapted to ensure good storage condition; protection from adverse weather conditions; separate earmarked areas in same warehouse for quarantine status; separate sampling area; segregation for storage of rejected, recalled or returned materials; safe and secure areas for NDPS and hazardous substances; safe storage of printed packaging material; separate dispensing areas for Beta lactum, sex hormones, cytotoxic substances and other special categories; regular checks and rodent control.

- **Sterile Products**

  Separate enclosed area with air locks; air supply through HEPA filters; routine microbial counts; laminar flow cabinets availability and access restricted only to authorized persons.

- **Working Space**

  Adequate space for orderly placement of equipment and material; and separate storage area for raw material "under test", "approved" and "rejected". The pipe-work, electrical fittings and ventilation openings should be properly designed.

- **Health, Clothing and Sanitation of Workers**

  The workers should be free from contagious diseases. It covers regular medical check-up facilities; proper toilet facility at a distance; personal cupboards and change room for workers.

- **Medical Services**

  First-aid facility; medical examination of workers and all other staff at the time of recruitment; periodic medical check-up of all staff members once in a year; services of physicians available at short notice, proper facilities for vaccinations, etc.

- **Sanitation in Manufacturing Premises**

  No accumulated waste; no dust particles as far as possible; proper disinfection and cleaning of premises and no stagnant water. The manufacturing premises should be used for specific purpose for which it is designed.

- **Equipment**

  Properly installed to achieve operational efficiency; good quality equipment to be used. The equipment used should be such to facilitate through cleaning; prevent physical and chemical change through contact and minimize contamination. The written instructions for utilization of equipment be provided and accuracy, precision should be maintained.

- **Raw Materials**

  Properly identified; analyzed; containers of raw materials inspected for any damage; stored at optimum temperature; labeled properly; systematically sampled by quality control personnel; tested for compliance of required standards; released from quarantine by quality control personnel through written instructions; and rejected materials destroyed or returned back to the supplier.

- **Personnel Manufacture**

  Under direct supervision of competent technical staff; separate Head for Q.C. laboratory; qualified and experienced personnel for Quality

Assurance and Quality Control Operations; labeling; quarantine and storage; batch numbering; testing, records of analysis; equipment assembly and calibration; maintenance; cleaning and sanitation; personnel; pest control; complaints, and recalls made and returns received.

- **Manufacturing Operations and Controls**

  Competent technical staff supervision for weighing, measuring and other operations; nonsterile products free from *E. coli* and *Salmonella* microbes; conspicuously labelled with name, batch number, and other details; cross contamination avoided; and all process controls checked under master formula.

- **Reprocessing and Recovery**

  The reason for reprocessing should be specified, corrective measures for recovery should be spelt out only if permitted in Master Formula.

- **Product Containers**

  Compliance with pharmacopeial requirements; cleaning procedures and sterilization procedure should be properly followed. There should be written schedule for programs for cleaning of container. When bottles are not dried after washing, deionized water is used for rinsing.

- **Labels and Other Printed Materials**

  Stored properly and separately; used as and when required and should not be inter-mixed.

- **Distribution Records**

  Records properly maintained; records of complaints, adverse reactions and other reactions from consumers are also maintained.

- **Quality Control System**

  Detailed instructions for quality control of raw materials and finished product; quality control for packaging and labeling; adequacy of storage, quality control procedure revised as and when possible and qualitative examination of returned products.

1.1.5   PART II: Plant and Equipment (Salient Features)

The Part II of Schedule M gives the details of the plant and equipment required for manufacture, quality control and quality assurance of different dosage forms. The specifications of equipl!1ents are also indicated. The details of requirements are categorized into 11 groups.

1.1.5.1 External Preparations: It covers ointments, emulsions, lotions, solutions, pastes, creams, dusting powders and other identical preparations.

(a) **Minimum area:** 30 square meters for basic installation and 10 square meters for ancillary area.

(b) **Requirements:** Mixing and storage tanks, jacketed kettles of different types, electric mixer, planetary mixer, colloid mill, triple roller mill, liquid and tube filling equipments, etc.

1.1.5.2 Oral Liquid Preparations: It covers syrups, elixirs, emulsions and suspensions.

(a) **Minimum area:** 30 square meters for basic installation -and 10 square meters for ancillary area;

(b) **Requirements:** SS mixing and storage tanks, jacketed kettles of different types, electric stirrer, electric colloidal mill, emulsifier, filtration equipment, bottle filling machine, cap sealing machine, deionizer or water distillation unit, clarity testing unit, etc.

1.1.5.3 Tablets: For effective production, tablet production department is divided into four sections

Mixing, granulation and drying section

Tablet compression section

Packaging section (strip/blister)

Coating section

(a) **Minimum area:** A minimum of 60 square meters for basic installation and 20 square meters for ancillary area for un-coated tablets. For coated tablet, additional area of 30 square meters for coating section and 10 square meters for ancillary area.

(b) **Requirements:** Disintegrator, sifter, powder mixer, mass mixer, planetary mixer, rapid mixer granulator, granulator, hot air oven, weighing machines, compression machine (single, multi-punch, rotary), punches and dies storage cabinets, table de-duster, table inspection unit/belt, dissolution test apparatus, single pan balance, hardness tester, friability and disintegration test apparatus, strip/blister packaging machine, leak test apparatus, tablet counter, jacketed kettles of different types, SS coating pan, polishing pan, weighing balance, exhaust system and vacuum dust collector, air-conditioning system (wherever applicable), etc.

1.1.5.4 Powders

(a) **Area:** Minimum 30 square meters; additional room for actual blending

(b) **Requirements:** Disintegrator, electric mixer, sifter, SS vessels and scoops of suitable sizes, filling equipment, weighing balance, etc.

1.1.5.5 Capsules

(a) **Area:** A separate enclosed area, suitably air-conditioned and dehumidified. A minimum area of 25 square meters for basic installation and 10 square meters for ancillary area each for penicillin and non-penicillin section.

(b) **Requirements (for hard gelatin capsules):** Electrical mixing and blending equipment, capsule filling units (semiautomatic and automatic), capsules counters, weighing balance, disintegration test apparatus, capsule polishing equipment, etc.

1.1.5.6 Surgical Dressings

(a) **Area:** Minimum 30 square meters for basic installation; for medicated dressing additional room required.

(b) **Requirements:** Rolling, staining, cutting, folding and pressing machines; mixing tanks, hot air oven, steam sterilizer, work tables, etc.

1.1.5.7 Ophthalmic Preparations

It includes eye-ointment, eye lotions and other preparations for external use. Separate enclosed areas with air-lock arrangements required.

(a) **Area:** Minimum 25 square meters for basic installation and 10 square meters for ancillary area.

(b) **Requirements:** Hot air ovens, jacketed kettles of different types, colloid mill, ointment mill, SS-mixing and storage tanks; tube washing, drying, cleaning and filling machines; automatic vial washing machine, vial drying machines, sintered glass funnels, autoclave, liquid filling equipment, laminar flow units, air conditioning and dehumidification arrangement. rubber bung washing machine, etc.

1.1.5.8 Pessaries and Suppositories

(a) **Area:** Minimum 25 square meters for basic installation

(b) **Requirements:** Mixing, pouring and molding equipments; weighing devices. For pessaries manufactured by granulation and compression, requirements shall be as given under "tablet".

1.1.5.9 Inhalers and Vitrallae

(a) **Area:** Minimum 25 square meters for basic installation.

(b) **Requirements**: Mixing, graduated delivery and sealing equipments.

1.1.5.10 Repacking of Drugs and Pharmaceuticals

(a) **Area:** Minimum 30 square meters for basic installation. Exhaust system be provided in case of operations involving floating particles.

(b) **Requirements:** Weighing, measuring and filling equipments; powder disintegrator, electrically operated powder sifter, electric sealing machine, SS scoops and vessels, etc.

1.1.5.11 Parenteral Preparations: The whole operation of manufacture (small volume injectables and large volume parenterals) in glass and plastic preparations are divided in separate areas/rooms.

A. **Parenteral Preparations in glass containers:** It includes areas for water management, containers, closures preparation, solution preparation, filling, capping, sealing, sterilization, quarantine, visual inspection and packaging.

(a) **Area:** Minimum 150 square meters for basic installation and 100 square meters for ancillary area for small volume injectables.

(b) **Requirements:** Distillation unit, deionized water unit, thermostatically controlled water storage tank, transfer pumps, SS service lines for carrying water, automatic rotary ampoule/vial/bottle washing machine, automatic closures, washing machine, dryer, double ended sterilizer; storage equipment for ampoules, vials, bottles and closures, SS benches/stools, dust proof storage cabinets, mixing SS tanks, portable stirrer, filtration equipment, transfer pumps, automatic ampoule/vial/bottle filling, capping, sealing machines under laminar air flow work station; gas lines for nitrogen, oxygen and carbon dioxide; steam sterilizer, hot air sterilizer, storage cabinets, visual inspection units, batch coding, machine labeling unit, pressure leak test apparatus, etc.

For large volume parenterals the minimum area required is 150 square meters each for basic installation and ancillary area.

B. **Parenteral Preparations in Plastic Containers by Form - FiII-Seal/Blow, FiII- Seal technology**

The operational activities are in separate areas for water management, solution preparation, container-moulding-cum-filling, sealing, sterilization, quarantine, visual inspection and packaging.

(a) **Area:** Minimum 250 square meters for basic installation and 150 square meters for ancillary area. Areas for formulations meant for external and internal uses shall be separately provided. A minimum of 100 squares meters be provided for packaging materials for large volume parenterals.

(b) Requirements: Deionized water treatment unit, distillation unit (multi-column with heat exchangers), thermostatically controlled water storage tank, transfer pumps, storage tanks, solution preparation tanks, transfer pumps, cartridge and membrane filters, sterile form fill-seal machine, plastic granules feeding device, super-heated steam sterilizer, adequate number of platforms, racks for storage, visual inspection unit, pressure leak test apparatus, batch coding machine, labelling unit, etc.

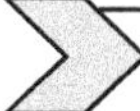 **1.2   TQM**

In order to understand "Total quality management", first we have to understand what does 'Quality' actually mean?

'Quality' is generally referred to a parameter which decides the inferiority or superiority of a product or service. It is a measure of goodness to understand how a product meets its specifications. Usually, when the expression "quality" is used, we think in the terms of an excellent product or service that meets or even exceeds our expectations. These expectations are based on the price and the intended use of the goods or services. In simple words, when a product or service exceeds our expectations, we consider it to be of good quality. Therefore, it is somewhat of an intangible expression based upon perception.

1.2.1 Definition of TQM

Total Quality Management is defined as a customer-oriented process and aims for continuous improvement of business operations. It ensures that all allied works (particularly work of employees) are toward the common goals of improving product quality or service quality, as well as enhancing the production process or process of rendering of services. However, the emphasis is put on fact-based decision making, with the use of performance metrics to monitor progress.

1.2.2 The Key Principles of Total Quality Management

Commitment from the management:

- Plan (drive, direct)
- Do (deploy, support, and participate)
- Check (review)
- Act (recognize, communicate, revise)

Employee Empowerment

- Training
- Excellence team

- Measurement and recognition
- Suggestion scheme

Continuous Improvement

- Systematic measurement
- Excellence teams
- Cross-functional process management
- Attain, maintain, improve standards

Customer Focus

- Partnership with Suppliers
- Service relationship with internal customers
- Customer-driven standards
- Never compromise quality

1.2.3   Benefits of Total Quality Management

The benefits arising from the implementation of a Total Quality Management in an organization are:

- This will increase the awareness of quality culture within the organization.
- A special emphasis on teamwork will be achieved.

1.2.4 Beliefs about Total Quality Management

Following are the universal Total Quality Management beliefs:

- Satisfaction of the customer/owner is the measure of quality.
- Everyone is an owner.
- Continuous Quality improvement must be there.
- Analysis of the processes is the key to quality improvement.
- Constant TQM is not possible without consistent, active and enabling leadership by managers at all levels.
- It is important to incessantly improve quality of the products and services which we are supposed to provide to our customers/owners.

1.2.5   The 8 Primary Elements of TQM

Total quality management can be summarized as a management system for a customer-focused organization that involves all employees in continual improvement. It uses strategy, data, and effective communications to integrate the quality discipline into the culture and activities of the organization. Many of these concepts are present in modern Quality

Management Systems, the successor to TQM. Here are the 8 principles of total quality management:

A. Customer-focused

The customer ultimately determines the level of quality. No matter what an organization does to foster quality improvement-training employees, integrating quality into the design process, upgrading computers or software, or buying new measuring tools-the customer determines whether the efforts were worthwhile.

B. Total employee involvement

All employees participate in working toward common goals. Total employee commitment can only be obtained after fear has been driven from the workplace, when empowerment has occurred, and management has provided the proper environment. High-performance work systems integrate continuous improvement efforts with normal business operations. Self-managed work teams are one form of empowerment.

C. Process-centered

A fundamental part of TQM is a focus on process thinking. A process is a series of steps that take inputs from suppliers (internal or external) and transforms them into outputs that are delivered to customers (again, either internal or external). The steps required to carry out the process are defined, and performance measures are continuously monitored in order to detect unexpected variation.

D. Integrated system

Although an organization may consist of many different functional specialties often organized into vertically structured departments, it is the horizontal processes interconnecting these functions that are the focus of TQM.

Micro-processes add up to larger processes, and all processes aggregate into the business processes required for defining and implementing strategy. Everyone must understand the vision, mission, and guiding principles as well as the quality policies, objectives, and critical processes of the organization. Business performance must be monitored and communicated continuously.

An integrated business system may be modeled after the Baldrige National Quality Program criteria and/or incorporate the ISO 9000 standards. Every organization has a unique work culture, and it is virtually impossible to achieve excellence in its products and services unless a good quality culture has been fostered. Thus, an integrated system connects business improvement elements in an attempt to continually improve and exceed the expectations of customers, employees, and other stakeholders.

E. Strategic and systematic approach

A critical part of the management of quality is the strategic and systematic approach to achieving an organization's vision, mission, and goals. This process, called strategic planning or strategic management, includes the formulation of a strategic plan that integrates quality as a core component.

F. Continual improvement

A major thrust of TQM is continual process improvement. Continual improvement drives an organization to be both analytical and creative in finding ways to become more competitive and more effective at meeting stakeholder expectations.

G. Fact-based decision making

In order to know how well an organization is performing, data on performance measures are necessary. TQM requires that an organization continually collect and analyze data in order to improve decision making accuracy, achieve consensus, and allow prediction based on past history.

H. Communications

During times of organizational change, as well as part of day-to-day operation, effective communications play a large part in maintaining morale and in motivating employees at all levels. Communications involve strategies, method, and timeliness.

These elements are considered so essential to TQM that many organizations define them, in some format, as a set of core values and principles on which the organization is to operate. The methods for implementing this approach come from the teachings of such quality leaders as Philip B. Crosby, W. Edwards Deming, Armand V. Feigenbaum, Kaoru Ishikawa, and Joseph M. Juran.

1.2.6   Influences on The Total Quality Management Philosophy

The Philosophy of TQM was born out of the concepts developed by namely **four great gurus** of Quality management.

- W. Edwards Deming
- Joseph M Juran
- Armand V Feigenbaum
- Philip Crosby

Here is a short introduction to their concepts and how these contributed to Total Quality Management Philosophy that we have today.

W. Edwards Deming

Deming's argument was that quality that is achieved through a reduction in statistical variation improves competitive position as well as productivity.

He defined Quality as being the direct result of quality of design, quality of conformance and the quality of the sales and service function.

A great believer in measuring quality by direct statistical measurement against specification, the goal of quality improvement is to reduce variation.

He developed a set of 14 points for management that express these issues. His beliefs were that quality management and improvement were the responsibility of all employees in a company.

Deming also believed that managers must change and to develop partnerships with those at the operating level of the business, one of the key elements in the Total Quality Management Philosophy.

Joseph Juran

Juran was probably the greatest contributor to the Total Quality Management Philosophy.He developed his ten-point plan which is the backbone of TQM implementation nowadays.

The Juran Method:
1. Build awareness of the need and opportunity for improvement
2. Set goals for improvement
3. Organize to reach the goals
4. Provide training
5. Carry out projects to solve problems
6. Report progress
7. Give recognition
8. Communicate results
9. Keep the score
10. Maintain momentum by making annual improvement part of the regular system and processes of the company.

Juran defined Quality as being "Fitness for Use" and really emphasized the cost of quality.

He believed that it was important to take management structure as a starting point and to build the quality improvement program from that baseline.

Armand Feigenbaum

Feigenbaum was the originator of the term "Total Quality Control". He believed that significant quality improvement could only be achieved by the participation of everyone in the organisation.

Fire-fighting quality management should be replaced with clear, customer-oriented quality management which the employees understand and can commit themselves to.

Feigenbaum believed that the goal of Quality improvement was to reduce the total cost of quality to as low a percentage as possible.

Philip Crosby

Philip Crosby's argument is that higher quality will ultimately reduce costs. He defined Quality as being the "Conformance to Requirements".

He developed a program with 14 steps that has the focus of changing an organization using action plans for their implementation.

His absolute beliefs were that

1. Quality means conformance and not elegance
2. It is always cheaper to do a job right first-time round
3. The only performance indicator is the cost of quality
4. The only performance standard is Zero Defects

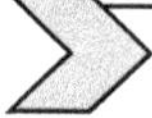 ## 1.3   ICH Guidelines

ICH is the "International Conference on Harmonization of Technical Requirements for Registration of Pharmaceuticals for Human Use" was established in 1990 as a tripartite venture representing regulatory bodies and research-based industry. ICH is a joint initiative involving both regulators and research-based industry representatives of the EU, Japan and the US in scientific and technical discussions of the testing procedures required to assess and ensure the safety, quality and efficacy of medicines.

The ICH Secretariat is based in Geneva. The biennial meetings and conferences of the ICH Steering Committee rotate between the EU, Japan, and the USA.

1.3.1   Objectives of ICH

- To increase international harmonization of technical requirements to ensure that safe, effective and high-quality medicines are developed.
- To harmonize technical requirements for registration or marketing approval.

- To develop and register pharmaceuticals in the most efficient and cost-effective manner.

- To promote public health.

- To prevent unnecessary duplication of clinical trials on humans.

- To minimize the use of animal testing without compromising safety and effectiveness of drug.

1.3.2 Purpose of ICH

- To promote international harmonization by bringing together representatives from the three ICH regions (EU, Japan and USA)

- To discuss and establish common guidelines.

- To make information available on ICH, ICH activities and ICH guidelines to any country or company that requests the information

- To promote a mutual understanding of regional initiatives in order to facilitate harmonization processes related to ICH guidelines regionally and globally

- To strengthen the capacity of drug regulatory authorities and industry to utilize them.

1.3.3 Participants of ICH

- ICH is comprised of representatives from six parties that represent the regulatory bodies and research-based industry in the European Union, Japan and the USA.

- In Japan, the members are the Ministry of Health, Labour and Welfare (MHLW), and the Japan Pharmaceutical Manufacturers Association (JPMA).

- In Europe, the members are the European Union (EU), and the European Federation of Pharmaceutical Industries and Associations (EFPIA).

- In the USA, the members are the Food and Drug Administration (FDA), and the Pharmaceutical Research and Manufacturers of America (PhRMA).

- Additional members include Observers from the World Health Organization (WHO), European Free Trade Association (EFTA), and Canada. The Observers represent non-ICH countries and regions.

1.3.4 ICH Structure

The ICH structure consists of the ICH Steering Committee, ICH Coordinators, ICH Secretariat and ICH Working Groups.

1.3.4.1 ICH Steering Committee

The Steering Committee is the body that governs the ICH, determines the policies and procedures for ICH, selects topics for harmonization and monitors the progress of harmonization initiatives. Each of the six ICH parties has two seats on the ICH Steering Committee.

1.3.4.2 ICH Coordinators

The Coordinators are fundamental to the smooth running of the ICH and are nominated by each of the six parties. An ICH Coordinator acts as the main contact point with the ICH Secretariat.

1.3.4.3 ICH Secretariat

The Secretariat is primarily concerned with preparations for, and documentation of, meetings of the Steering Committee as well as coordination of preparations for Working Group and Discussion Group meetings. Information on ICH Guidelines and the general ICH process can be obtained from the ICH Secretariat.

1.3.4.4 ICH Working Group

Depending on the type of harmonization activity needed, the Steering Committee will endorse the establishment of one of three types of working group i.e., Expert Working Group (EWG), Implementation Working Group (IWG) or Informal Working Group.

1.3.5 Steps in the ICH Process

Step-1: Drafts are prepared and circulated through many revisions until a "final harmonised draft" is completed

Step-2: This draft is signed by the EWG as the agreed upon draft and forwarded to the Steering Committee for signing which signifies acceptance for consultation by each of the six co-sponsors

Step-3: The three regulatory sponsors initiate their normal consultation process to receive comments.

Step-4: is reached when the Steering Committee agrees that there is sufficient scientific consensus on the technical issues. This endorsement is based on the signatures from the three regulatory parties to ICH affirming that the Guideline is recommended for adoption by the regulatory bodies of the three regions.

Step-5: The process is complete when the guidelines are incorporated into national or regional internal procedures (implementation in the 3 ICH regions).

1.3.6   Overview of QSEM

"Quality" Topics, i.e., those relating to chemical and pharmaceutical Quality Assurance (Stability Testing, Impurity Testing, etc.)

Efficacy" Topics, i.e., those relating to clinical studies in human subject (Dose Response Studies, Good Clinical Practices, etc.)

Safety" Topics, i.e., those relating to in vitro and in vivo pre-clinical studies (Carcinogenicity Testing, Genotoxicity Testing, etc.)

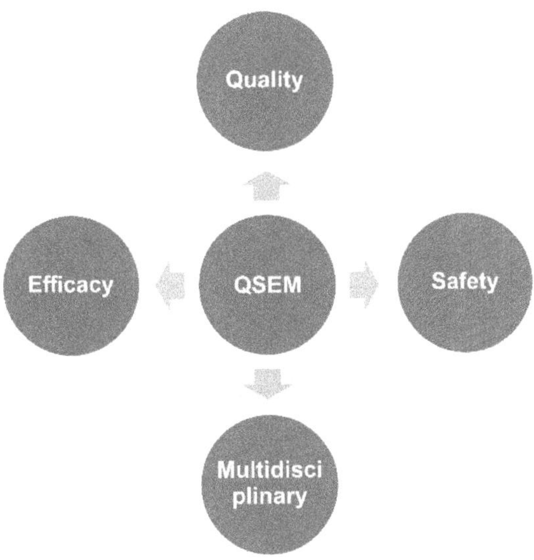

Multidisciplinary" Topics, i.e., cross-cutting Topics which do not fit uniquely into one of the above categories.

1.3.7   Quality Guidelines

"Quality" Topics, i.e., those relating to chemical and pharmaceutical Quality Assurance (Stability Testing, Impurity Testing, etc.)

Q1A-Q1F---STABILITY

OBJECTIVE OF STABILITY TESTING- "...... to provide evidence on how the quality of a drug substance or drug product varies with time under the influence of a variety of environmental factors such as temperature, humidity & light, & enables recommended storage conditions, re-test periods & shelf lives to be established"

Variables affecting the stability-

- Formulation
- Packaging
- Site and method of
- manufacture API Finished product
- Batch size
- Batch to batch variability Process validation Quality risk management
- Container labelling
- Changes to product

1.3.8   Adverse Effects of Instability of Drugs

- Loss of active drug (e.g. aspirin hydrolysis, oxidation of adrenaline)
- Loss of vehicle (e.g. evaporation of water from o/w creams, evaporation of alcohol from alcoholic mixtures)
- Loss of content uniformity (e.g. creaming of emulsions, impaction of suspensions)
- Loss of elegance (e.g. fading of tablets and colored solutions)
- Reduction in bioavailability (e.g. ageing of tablets resulting in a change in dissolution profile)
- Production of potential toxic materials (e.g. breakdown products from drug degradation

1.3.9   Types of Stability

- **CHEMICAL**: Each active ingredient retains its chemical integrity and labeled potency within the specified limit.
- **PHYSICAL**: The physical stability properties includes appearance, palatability, uniformity, dissolution and suspend ability are retained.
- **MICROBIOLOGICAL**: Sterility or resistance to microbial growth is retained according to specified requirement.
- **THERAPEUTIC**: Therapeutic activity remains unchanged.
- **TOXICOLOGIC**: No significant increase in toxicity occurs.

1.3.10   Stability Testing

Development studies-

- Characterize compatibility with common excipients.
- Characterize stability profile of API (e.g. susceptibility to acid, base, light, oxygen etc)
- Characterize stability profile of early formulations (Especially susceptibility to heat, humidity & light) Confirmatory studies.
- Long term & accelerated studies on the product as it is to be registered.

1.3.11   Q1A (R2): Stability Testing of New Drug Substances and Products

The purpose of stability testing is to provide evidence on how the quality of a drug substance or drug product varies with time under the influence of a variety of environmental factors such as temperature, humidity, and light, and to establish a re-test period for the drug substance or a shelf life for the drug product.

1.3.11.1 General

Information on the stability of the drug substance is an integral part of the systematic approach to stability evaluation.

1.3.11.2 Stress Testing

Main tool that predicts the stability problems

- Foundation for developing and validating analytical methods.
- When available, it is acceptable to provide relevant data published in the scientific literature to support the identified degradation pathways and products.

1.3.11.3 Roll of Stress Testing

- Stress testing of the active substance can help in
- Identification of degradants
- Identification of degradation pathways
- Determination of which type(s) of stress affect the molecule: Photo-stability High Temperature Low Temperature Oxidation pH extremes Water

Oxidation

- Typically done by placing the drug substance in aqueous solution of hydrogen peroxide.
- Goal is significant degradation (typically 10-30% of API) Can identify degradants Determine whether protective packaging is required Determine if an antioxidant should be considered for the drug product formulation.

pH

- Typically done by adding drug substance to buffered aqueous solutions at pH values from 1-10
- Decide if the molecule will survive passage through the stomach
- Is enteric coating necessary?
- the drug be given by injection?

1.3.11.4 Selection of Batches

- Data from formal stability studies should be provided on at least three primary batches of the active substance.

- The batches should be manufactured to a minimum of pilot scale by the same synthetic route as, and using a method of manufacture and procedure that simulates the final process to be used for, production batches.

1.3.11.5 Container and Closure System

The stability studies should be conducted on the active substance packaged in a container closure system that is the same as or simulates the packaging proposed for storage and distribution.

1.3.11.6 Specification

- Stability studies should include testing of those attributes of the drug substance that are susceptible to change during storage and are likely to influence quality, safety, and/or efficacy.
- The testing should cover, as appropriate, the physical, chemical, biological, and microbiological attributes. e.g. appearance, assay, degradation.

1.3.11.7 Testing Frequency

For long term studies:

Year 1: every 3 months

Year 2: every 6 months

Subsequent years: annually

At accelerated storage conditions: (6 months study)

Minimum three points including t_0 and t_{final}

e.g. 0 (initial)   3   6 (final)

At intermediate storage conditions: (12 months study)

Four points including t_0 and t_{final}

e.g. 0 (initial)   6   9   12 (final)

1.3.11.8 Storage Condition

A drug substance should be evaluated:

- To test its thermal stability
- Its sensitivity to moisture (if applicable)
- The long-term testing (minimum of 12 months) on at least 3 primary batches at the time of submission and
- Should be continued for a period of time sufficient to cover the proposed re-test period.

1.3.11.9 General Case

Study	Storage condition	Minimum time period covered by data at submission
Long Term* (Ambient)	25° C ± 2° C 60% RH ± 5%	12 months
Intermediate** (controlled)	30° C ± 2° C 65% RH ± 5%	6 months
Accelerated	40° C ± 2° C 75% RH ± 5%	6 months

1.3.11.10 Storage in Refrigerator

Study	Storage condition	Minimum time period covered by data at submission
Long Term	5° C ± 3° C	12 months
Accelerated	25° C ± 2° C 60% RH ± 5%	6 months

1.3.11.11 Storage in a Freezer

Study	Storage condition	Minimum time period covered by data at submission
Long Term	-20° C ± 5° C	12 months

1.3.11.12 Evaluation

- Minimum of 3 batches of drug substance is tested.
- The degree of variability of individual batches affects the confidence that a future production batch will remain within specification throughout the assigned re-test period.
- The analyst must find batch-to-batch variability & if it is small than only it is accepted & it can be done by different statistical test's (P value for level of significance for rejection).
- Where the data show so little degradation and so little variability then it is normally unnecessary to go through the statistical analysis; providing a justification for the omission should be sufficient.

1.3.11.13 Statement/Labeling

- A storage statement should be established for the labelling based on the stability evaluation of the active substance.
- Where applicable, specific instructions should be provided, particularly for active substances that cannot tolerate freezing. Terms such as "ambient conditions" or "room temperature" must be avoided.

1.3.11.14 Stability-Indicating Quality Parameter

Stability studies should include testing of those attributes of the Drug product that are susceptible to change during storage and are likely to influence quality, safety and/or efficacy. For instance, in case of tablets: appearance hardness friability moisture content dissolution time degradants assay microbial purity.

1.13.11.15 Accelerated Stability

- This stability study run under more stressful conditions than expected for long term storage to account for any changes outside the label storage conditions.

- The goal is to get a quick understanding of what may be expected from a long-term study.

Q1B: Photostability Testing of New Drug Substances and Products

Give guidance on the basic testing protocol required to evaluate the light sensitivity and stability of new drugs and products.

Q1C: Stability Testing for New Dosage Forms

Gives guidelines for new formulations of already approved medicines and defines the circumstances under which reduced stability data can be accepted.

Q1D: Bracketing and Matrixing Designs for Stability

Testing of New Drug Substances and Products

Q1E: Evaluation of Stability Data

This guideline addresses the evaluation of stability data that should be submitted in registration applications for new molecular entities and associated drug products. The guideline provides recommendations on establishing shelf lives for drug substances and drug products intended for storage at or below "room temperature".

Q1F: Stability Data Package for Registration Applications in Climatic Zones III and IV

Describes harmonized global stability testing requirements in order to facilitate access to medicines by reducing the number of different storage conditions. WHO conducted a survey amongst their member states to find consensus on 30°C/65% RH as the longterm storage conditions for hot-dry and hot-humid regions.

1.3.12 Q2-Analytical validation

Q2(R1): Validation of Analytical Procedures: Text and Methodology

- The objective of validation of an analytical procedure is to demonstrate that it is suitable for its intended purpose

- Gives validation parameters needed for a variety of analytical methods.

- It also discusses the characteristics that must be considered during the validation of the analytical

- Procedures 18 Types of Analytical Procedures to be validated are:

  - Identification tests;

  - Quantitative tests for impurities content;

  - Limit tests for the control of impurities;

  - Quantitative tests of the active moiety in samples of drug substance or drug product or other selected components in the drug product.

- Typical validation characteristics of analytical procedures are; Accuracy, Precision (Repeatability, Intermediate Precision), Specificity, Detection Limit, Quantitation Limit, Linearity, Range.

1.3.13 Q3A- Q3D----Impurities

Q3A(R2): Impurities in New Drug Substances

- The guideline addresses the chemistry and safety aspects of impurities, including the listing of impurities, threshold limit, identification and quantification.

- Classification of Impurities: are of 3 types

- Organic impurities (process- and drug-related)

- Inorganic impurities

- Residual solvents

Q3B(R2): Impurities in New Drug Products

Q3C(R4): Impurities: Guideline for Residual Solvents

- Benzene   2 ppm
- Carbon tetrachloride   4 ppm
- Dichloromethane   5 ppm
- Dichloroethane   8 ppm
- Acetonitrile   410 ppm
- Chloroform   60 ppm

- Chlorobenzene   360 ppm
- Formamide, Hexane   290 ppm
- Toulene   890 ppm
- Pyridine   200 pm
- Nitromethane   50 ppm
- Methanol   3000 ppm

1.3.14 Q4: Pharmacopoeias

Q4A: Pharmacopeial Harmonization

Q4B: Evaluation and Recommendation of Pharmacopeial Texts for Use in the ICH Regions

This document describes a process for the evaluation and recommendation given by the Q4B Expert Working Group (EWG) for selecting pharmacopeial texts to facilitate their recognition by regulatory authorities for use, interchangeable in the ICH regions.

- Annex 1: Evaluation and Recommendation of Pharmacopeial Texts for Use in the ICH Regions on Residue on Ignition/Sulphated Ash
- Annex 2: Test for Extractable Volume of Parenteral Preparations
- Annex 3: Test for Particulate Contamination: Sub-Visible Particles
- Annex 4A: Microbiological Examination of Non-Sterile Products: Microbial Enumeration Tests
- Annex 4B: Microbiological Examination of Non-Sterile Products: Tests for Specified Micro-organisms
- Annex 4C: Microbiological Examination of Non-Sterile Products: Acceptance Criteria for Pharmaceutical Preparations and Substances for Pharmaceutical Use
- Annex 5: Disintegration Test
- Annex 6: Uniformity of Dosage Units
- Annex 7: Dissolution Test
- Annex 8: Sterility Test
- Annex 9: Tablet Friability
- Annex 10: Polyacrylamide Gel Electrophoresis
- Annex 11: Capillary Electrophoresis
- Annex 12: Analytical Sieving
- Annex 13: Bulk Density and Tapped Density of Powders
- Annex14: Bacterial Endotoxins Test

1.3.15 Q5A-Q5E---Quality of Biotechnological Products

Q5A(R1): Viral Safety Evaluation of Biotechnology Products Derived from Cell Lines of Human or Animal Origin

- This document is concerned with testing and evaluation of the viral safety of biotechnology products derived from cell lines of human or animal origin (i.e., mammalian, avian, insect)

- The objective is to provide a general framework for virus testing experiments for the evaluation of virus clearance and the design of viral tests and clearance evaluation studies. Three principal, complementary approaches have evolved to control the potential viral contamination of biotechnology products:

    (a) selecting and testing cell lines and other raw materials, including media components, for the

    (b) absence of undesirable viruses which may be infectious and/or pathogenic for humans;

    (c) Testing the capacity of the processes to clear infectious viruses;

    (d) testing the product at appropriate steps for absence of contaminating infectious viruses.

Q5B: Quality of Biotechnological Products: Analysis of the Expression Construct in Cells

Used for Production of r-DNA Derived Protein Products

- This document presents guidance regarding the characterization of the expression construct for the production of recombinant DNA protein products in eukaryotic and prokaryotic cells.

- Expression construct should be analyzed using nucleic acid techniques.

Q5C: Quality of Biotechnological Products: Stability Testing of Biotechnological/Biological Products

Q5D: Derivation and Characterization of Cell Substrates Used for Production of Biotechnological/Biological Products

- The objective of this guideline is to provide broad guidance on appropriate standards for cell substrates.

Q5E: Comparability of Biotechnological/ Biological Products Subject to Changes in Their Manufacturing Process

- The objective of this document is to provide principles for assessing the comparability of biotechnological/ biological products before and after changes are made in the manufacturing process for the drug substance or drug product.

- Therefore, this guideline is intended to assist in the collection of relevant technical information which serves as evidence that the manufacturing process changes will not have an adverse impact on the quality, safety and efficacy of the drug product.

1.3.16 Q6: Specifications for New Drug Substances and Products

- Bulk drug substance and final product specifications are key parts of the core documentation for world-wide product license applications.

- This leads to conflicting standards for the same product, increased expenses and opportunities for error as well as a potential cause for interruption of product supply.

Q6A: Specifications: Test Procedures and Acceptance Criteria for New Drug Substances and New Drug Products: Chemical Substances

- The main objective of this guideline is to establish a single set of global specifications for new drug substances and new drug products.

- A specification is defined as a list of tests, references to analytical procedures, and appropriate acceptance criteria, which are numerical limits, ranges

- This guideline addresses specifications, i.e., those tests, procedures, and acceptance criteria which play a major role in assuring the quality of the new drug substance and new drug product during shelf life.

Q6B: Specifications: Test Procedures and Acceptance Criteria for Biotechnological/Biological Products

- This document provides guidance on justifying and setting specifications for proteins and polypeptides which are derived from recombinant or non-recombinant cell cultures.

- A valid biological assay to measure the biological activity should be provided by the manufacturer.

- Examples of procedures used to measure biological activity include:
  - Animal-based biological assays, which measure an organism's biological response to the product;
  - Cell culture-based biological assays, which measure biochemical or physiological response at the cellular level;
  - Biochemical assays, which measure biological activities such as enzymatic reaction rates or biological responses induced by immunological interactions.

1.3.17 Q7: Good Manufacturing Practice Guide for Active Pharmaceutical Ingredients

- The main objective of this guideline is that to maintain the quality of the active pharmaceutical ingredients
- Personnel
- Buildings and Facilities
- Process equipment
- Documentation and Records

1.3.18 Q8(R2): Pharmaceutical Development

- This guideline is intended to provide guidance on the contents of Pharmaceutical Development of drug products
- The aim of pharmaceutical development is to design a quality product and its manufacturing process to consistently deliver the intended performance of the product.
- The Pharmaceutical Development section also describe the type of dosage form and the formulation that are suitable for the intended use.
- *Q8 gives information about Drug Substance, Excipients,* Container Closure System.

1.3.19 Q9: Quality Risk Management

- The purpose of this document is to offer a systematic approach to quality risk management.
- This guideline provides principles and tools for quality risk management that can be applied to all aspects of pharmaceutical quality including development, manufacturing, distribution; and the inspection and submission/review processes throughout the lifecycle of drug substances and drug (medicinal) products, biological and biotechnological products, including the use of raw materials, solvents, excipients, packaging and labeling materials.

Principles of Quality Risk Management

Two primary principles of quality risk management are:

- The evaluation of the risk to quality should be based on scientific knowledge and ultimately link to the protection of the patient; and
- The level of effort and documentation of the quality risk management process should be commensurate with the level of risk.

1.3.20 Q10: Pharmaceutical Quality System

- This document establishes a new ICH tripartite guideline describing a model for an effective quality management system for the pharmaceutical industry, referred to as the Pharmaceutical Quality System.

- Comprehensive model for an effective pharmaceutical quality system is based on International Standards Organization (ISO) quality concepts, includes applicable Good Manufacturing Practice (GMP) regulations.

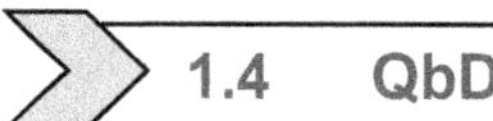

1.4   QbD

Pharmaceutical industry is moving towards quality. Many pharmaceutical companies have used several Quality Management System (QMS) for instance ISO 9001. Design process has one of the most important factors that contributing in pharmaceutical product quality. The pharmaceutical industry is used the concept of Quality by Design (QbD) to apply science-based manufacturing principles for new and existing products to assure quality of the formulation. In a first step, the QbD methodology is systematically used to establish the critical quality attribute identifies potentially critical input factor and these factors to define activities for process characterization. A process DOE was used to evaluate effects of the design factors on manufacturability and final product CQAs, and establish design space to ensure desired CQAs. Critical material and process parameters are linked to the critical quality attributes of the product. Experiments were designed with focus on critical material and process attributes. Quality by design is an essential part of the modern approach to pharmaceutical quality. The purpose of this article is to discuss the use of Quality by Design (QbD) in pharmaceuticals and describe how it can be used to ensure pharmaceutical quality. Process parameters and quality attributes were identified for each unit operation. The design space was established by the combined use of DOE, optimization and multivariate analysis to ensure desired CQAs. Multivariate analysis of all variables from the DOE batches was conducted to study relationships between the variables and to evaluate the impact of material attributes/process parameters on manufacturability and final product CQAs.

1.4.1 Pharmaceutical Quality by Design

QbD is a novel approach in pharmaceutical industry. It places more emphasis on continuous improvement rather than end-product testing. The pharma industry, however, is just beginning to experience the benefits of QbD.

The Quality by Design approach requires having a sound understanding of their product in the company. QbD makes certain that the product is of predictable and predefined quality. The adoption of QbD includes defining a target product quality profile; designing the manufacturing process from basic principles with a very good understanding of the mechanism involved (Design of Experiment); identifying critical quality areas, process parameters and potential sources of variability; and finally controlling manufacturing process to achieve the most consistent quality.

ICH Q8 defines quality as "The suitability of either a drug substance or drug product for its intended use. This term includes such attributes as the identity, strength, and purity." ICH Q6 emphasizes the role of specifications stating that "Specifications are critical quality standards that are proposed and justified by the manufacturer and approved by regulatory authorities 28." As per ICH Q8 defines that pharmaceutical Quality by Design (QbD) is "A systematic approach to development that begins with predefined objectives and emphasizes product and process understanding and process control, based on sound science and quality risk management." Pharmaceutical QbD is a systematic, scientific, risk-based, approach to pharmaceutical development that begins with predefined objectives. QbD identifies characteristics that are critical to quality and translates them into the attributes that the drug product should possess, and establishes how the critical process parameters can be varied to consistently produce a drug product with the desired characteristics.

Under the QbD approach, pharmaceutical quality for generic drugs is assured by understanding and controlling formulation and manufacturing variables. End product testing confirms the quality of the product and is not part of the manufacturing consistency or process control.

The specification for impurities assesses another important characteristic a drug product must have to ensure its safety. Under the QbD, the acceptance criterion of an impurity should be set based on its biological safety level instead of the actual batch data. The biological safety level is generally determined by safety studies although it may be also determined by toxicity studies. It should be noted that although there is a specification for a drug product under both the QbT and QbD paradigms, the roles that the specification plays are completely different. Under the QbT, each batch has to be tested against the specification to ensure its quality and manufacturing consistency. Under the QbD, batches may not be actually tested against the specification as the process understanding and/or process control provides sufficient evidences that the batches will meet the specification if tested, which allows the real time release of the batches. Further, the specification under the QbD is solely used for the confirmation of product quality, not manufacturing consistency and process control.

Combine prior knowledge with experiments to establish a design space or other representation of process understanding & establish a control strategy for the entire process that may include input material controls, process controls and monitors, design spaces around individual or multiple unit operations, and final product tests. The control strategy should encompass expected changes in scale and can be guided by a risk assessment. & continually monitor and update the process to assure consistent quality Design of experiments (DOE), risk assessment, and process analytical technology (PAT) are tools that may be used in the QbD process.

1.4.2   Identify Critical Quality Attributes, Process Parameters

The FDA has stated that "Quality by Design means that product and process performance characteristics are scientifically designed to meet specific objectives." As a direct consequence, one of the core tenets of Qbd is the requirement of detailed knowledge of the critical quality attributes (CQA) of the pharmaceutical product and the critical process parameters (CPPs) that can be used to control overall product quality. Gathering the raw data needed for this endeavor can be prohit time, labour, and cost intensive without employing Design of Experiment (DOE) approach, also known as Factorial Experiment Design (FED). Even with DOE, a significant number of samples need to be processed, which has created a need for next generation.

A pharmaceutical manufacturing process is usually comprised of a series of unit operations to produce the desired product. A unit operation is a discrete activity that involves physical changes, such as mixing, milling, granulation, drying, compaction, and coating. A physical, chemical or microbiological property or characteristic of an input or output material is defined as an attribute. Process parameters include the type of equipment and equipment settings, batch size, operating conditions (e.g., time, temperature, pressure, pH, and speed), and environmental conditions such as moisture. The quality and quantity of drug substance and excipients are considered as attributes of raw materials. During process development, raw materials, process parameters and quality attributes are investigated. The purpose of these studies is to determine the critical raw material attributes, process parameters and quality attributes for each process, and to establish any possible relationships among them. Critical quality attributes (CQA) are physical, chemical, biological, or microbiological property or characteristic that must be controlled directly or indirectly to ensure the quality of the product. Critical process parameters (CPP) are process inputs that have a direct and significant influence on critical quality attributes when they are varied within the regular operating range. Lists typical tablet manufacturing unit operations, process parameters, and quality attributes for solid dosage forms. It should be noted that the equipment maintenance, operator training, standard of operation (SOP) related to the specific product manufacturing, and facility supporting systems may link to product quality directly or indirectly.

Design of experiments (DOE) is a structured and organized method to determine the relationship among factors that influence outputs of a process. When DOE is applied to pharmaceutical process, factors are the raw material attributes (e.g., particle size) and process parameters (e.g., speed and time), while outputs are the critical quality attributes such as blend uniformity, tablet hardness, thickness, and friability. As each unit operation has many input and output variables as well as process parameters. DOE results can help identify optimal conditions, the critical factors that most influence CQAs Based on the acceptable range of CQAs, the design space of CPPs can be determined.

1.4.2.1 Critical Quality Attributes

ICH Q8 (R1) defines CQAs as physical, chemical, biological or microbiological properties or characteristics that should be within an appropriate limit, range, or distribution to ensure the desired product quality. CQA is used to describe both aspects of product performance and determinants of product performance. CQA is generally assumed to be an attribute of the final product, but it is also possible to indicate a CQA of an intermediate or a raw material.

1.4.2.2 Critical Process Parameters

Critical process parameter as any measurable input or output of a process step that must be controlled to achieve the desired product quality and process consistency. Process parameter be understood as referring to the input operating parameters (mixing speed, flow rate) and process state variables (temperature, pressure) of a process or unit operation. Under this definition, the state of a process depends on its CPPs and the CMAs of the input materials. Monitoring and controlling output material attributes can be a better control strategy than monitoring operating parameters especially for scale up. For example, a material attribute, such as moisture content, should have the same target value in the pilot and commercial processes. An operating parameter, such as air flow rate, would be expected to change as the process scale changes.

1.4.3   Essential Five-Step for Qbd for the Purpose of Product Development

Step I: Ascertaining Drug Product Objective(s)

The quality target product profile (QTPP) is a prospective summary of quality characteristics of the drug delivery product ideally achieved to ensure the desired quality, taking into account the safety and efficacy of the drug product. During drug product development, QTPP is embarked through brain storming among the team members cutting across multiple disciplines in the industry. Critical Quality Attributes (CQAs) are the physical, chemical, biological or microbiological characteristic of the product that should be within an appropriate limit, range or distribution to ensure the desired product quality. There are various types of CQAs associated with the drug products such as drug substance CQAs, excipients CQAs, packaging material CQAs, etc. The identification of prime CQAs from the QTPP is based on the severity of harm a patient may get plausibly owing to the product failure. Thus, after defining the QTPP, the CQAs which pragmatically epitomize the objective(s), are earmarked for the purpose.

Step II: Prioritizing Input Variables for Optimization

Material attributes (MAs) and process parameters (PPs) are considered as the independent input variables associated with a product and/or process, which directly influence the CQAs of the drug product. PPs can be of different types such as non-critical Process Parameters (non-CPPs), Unclassified Process Parameters (UPPs) and Critical Process Parameters (CPPs). Ishikawa-Fish bone diagram are used for establishment of cause-effect relationship among the input variables affecting the quality traits of the drug product. Figure 4 illustrates a typical cause-effect diagram highlighting the plausible causes of product variability and their impact on drug product CQAs. Figure 6 portrays the flow layout of overall risk assessment plan employing risk assessment and risk management for identifying the potential CMAs employing a prototype REM model. The low-resolution first-order experimental designs (e.g., fractional factorial, Plackett-Burman and Taguchi designs) are highly helpful for screening and factor influence studies. Before venturing into product or process optimization, prioritization of CMAs/CPPs using such QRM and/ or screening is obligatory

Step III: Design-guided Experimentation & Analysis

Response surface methodology is considered as a pivotal part of the entire QbD exercise for optimization of product and/or process variables discerned from the risk assessment and screening studies. The experimental designs help in mapping the responses on the basis of the studied objective(s), CQAs being explored, at high, medium or low levels of CMAs. Figure 7 diagrammatically enumerates the key experimental designs employed during QbD-based product development for response surface methodology and/or factor screening. Factorial, Box-Behnken, composite, optimal and mixture designs are the commonly used high resolution second-order designs employed for drug product optimization. Design matrix is a layout of experimental runs in matrix form generated by the chosen experimental design, to guide the drug delivery scientists. The drug formulations are experimentally prepared according to the design matrix and the chosen response variables are evaluated meticulously.

Step IV: Modelization & Validation of QbD Methodology

Modelization is carried out by selection of apt mathematical models like linear, quadratic and cubic models to generate the 2D and 3Dresponse surface to relate the response variables or CQAs with the input variables or CMAs/CPPs for identifying underlying interaction(s) among them. Multiple Linear Regression Analysis (MLRA), Partial Least Squares (PLS) analysis and Principal Component Analysis (PCA) are some of the key multivariate chemometric techniques employed for modelization to discern the factor-response relationship. Besides, the model diagnostic plots like perturbation charts, outlier plot, leverage plot, Cook's distance plot and Box-Cox plot are also helpful in unearthing the pertinent scientific, minutiae and interactions among the CMAs too. The search for optimum solution is accomplished through numerical and graphical optimization techniques like desirability function, canonical analysis, artificial neural network, brute-force methodology and overlay plot. Subsequent to the optimum search, the optimized formulation is located in the design and control spaces. Design space is a multidimensional combination of input variables (i.e., CMAs/CPPs) and out variable (i.e., CQAs) to discern the optimal solution with assurance of quality. Figure 9 illustrates the interrelationship among various spaces like, explorable, knowledge, design and control spaces. Usually in industrial milieu, a narrower domain of control space is construed from the design space for further implicit and explicit studies.

Step V: QbD Validation, Scale-up and Production

Validation of the QbD methodology is a crucial step that forecasts about the prognostic ability of the polynomial models studied. Various product and process parameters are selected from the experimental domain and evaluated as per the standard operating conditions laid down for the desired product and process related conditions carried out earlier, commonly termed as checkpoints or confirmatory runs. The results obtained from these checkpoints are then compared with the predicted ones through linear correlation plots and the residual plots to check any typical pattern like ascending or descending lines, cycles, etc. To corroborate QbD performance, the product or process is scaled-up through pilot-plant, exhibit and production scale, in an industrial milieu to ensure the reproducibility and robustness. A holistic and versatile "control strategy" is meticulously postulated for "continuous improvement" in accomplishing better quality of the finished product.

1.4.4   Software Usage during QbD

The merits of QbD techniques are galore and their acceptability upbeat. Putting such rational approaches into practice, however, usually involves a great deal of mathematical and statistical intricacies. Today, with the availability of powerful and economical hardware and that of the comprehensive QbD software, the erstwhile computational hiccups have been greatly simplified and streamlined. Figure 10 enlist the select computer software available commercially for carrying out QbD studies in industrial milieu. Pertinent computer software available for DoE optimization include Design-Expert®, Minitab®, MODDE®, Unscrambler®, JMP®, Statistica®, etc., are at the rescue, which usually provide interface guide at every step during the entire product development cycle. Software providing support for chemometric analysis through multivariate techniques like MNLRA, PCA, PLS, etc. encompass, MODDE®, Unscrambler®, SIMCA®, CODDESA®. For QRM execution using Fish-bone diagrams, REM and FMEA matrices during risk assessment studies, etc., software like, Minitab®, Risk®, Statgraphics, FMEA-Pro, iGrafx, etc., can be made use of.

1.5   ISO

The International Organization for Standardization (ISO), established in 1947, is an international organization of national standards bodies from more than 145 countries, with one body representing each country. ISO is based in Geneva, Switzerland. Its goal is to promote the development of standardization and related activities in the world; to facilitate the international exchange of goods and services; and to develop cooperation in intellectual, scientific, technological and economic activity. ISO's work results in international agreements, which are published as International Standards and other types of ISO documents.

1.5.1   Benefits of ISO

- ISO standards add value to all types of businesses and contribute for making the development, manufacturing, and supply of products and services more efficient, safer, and cleaner.

- They make trade between countries easier and fairer.

- ISO standards also serve to safeguard consumers and users of products and services in general as well as to make their lives simpler.

- The businesses that adopt international standards are increasingly free to compete in markets around the world.

- For customers, a product or service based on an international standard will be compatible with more products or services worldwide, which increases the number of choices available.

- Each ISO national committee can adopt an international standard. When the U.S. believes in the usefulness of a standard, that standard goes through an adoption process to make it an American National Standard. When an ISO standard has been adopted by the United States, the international community knows that the United States supports the content of that standard.

1.5.2 ISO 9000

ISO 9000 is defined as a set of international standards on quality management and quality assurance developed to help companies effectively document the quality system elements needed to maintain an efficient quality system. They are not specific to any one industry and can be applied to organizations of any size.

ISO 9000 can help a company satisfy its customers, meet regulatory requirements, and achieve continual improvement. It should be considered to be a first step or the base level of a quality system.

History

ISO 9000 was first published in 1987 by the International Organization for Standardization (ISO). The standards underwent major revisions in 2000 and 2008. The most recent versions of the standard, ISO 9000:2015 and ISO 9001:2015, were published in September 2015.

The ISO 9000:2000 revision had five goals:

1. Meet stakeholder needs
2. Be usable by all sizes of organizations
3. Be usable by all sectors
4. Be simple and clearly understood
5. Connect quality management system to business processes

ISO 9000:2015 principles of Quality Management

The ISO 9000:2015 and ISO 9001:2015 standards are based on seven quality management principles that senior management can apply to promote organizational improvement.

1. Customer focus

- Understand the needs of existing and future customers
- Align organizational objectives with customer needs and expectations

- Meet customer requirements
- Measure customer satisfaction
- Manage customer relationships
- Aim to exceed customer expectations
- Learn more about the customer experience and customer satisfaction

2. Leadership

- Establish a vision and direction for the organization
- Set challenging goals
- Model organizational values
- Establish trust
- Equip and empower employees
- Recognize employee contributions
- Learn more about leadership

3. Engagement of people

- Ensure that people's abilities are used and valued
- Make people accountable
- Enable participation in continual improvement
- Evaluate individual performance
- Enable learning and knowledge sharing
- Enable open discussion of problems and constraints
- Learn more about employee involvement

4. Process approach

- Manage activities as processes
- Measure the capability of activities
- Identify linkages between activities
- Prioritize improvement opportunities
- Deploy resources effectively
- Learn more about a process view of work and see process analysis tools

5. Improvement

- Improve organizational performance and capabilities
- Align improvement activities

- Empower people to make improvements
- Measure improvement consistently
- Celebrate improvements
- Learn more about approaches to continual improvement

6. Evidence-based decision making

- Ensure the accessibility of accurate and reliable data
- Use appropriate methods to analyze data
- Make decisions based on analysis
- Balance data analysis with practical experience
- See tools for decision making

7. Relationship management

- Identify and select suppliers to manage costs, optimize resources, and create value
- Establish relationships considering both the short and long term
- Share expertise, resources, information, and plans with partners
- Collaborate on improvement and development activities
- Recognize supplier successes
- Learn more about supplier quality and see resources related to managing the supply chain

1.5.3   ISO 14000

ISO 14000 is defined as a series of international environmental management standards, guides, and technical reports. The standards specify requirements for establishing an environmental management policy, determining environmental impacts of products or services, planning environmental objectives, implementing programs to meet objectives, and conducting corrective action and management review.

History

- The first environmental management system standard, BS 7750, was published in 1992 by the BSI group.
- In 1996, the International Organization for Standardization (ISO) created the ISO 14000 family of standards.
- ISO 14001 underwent revision in 2004.
- The current revision of ISO 14001 was published in September 2015.

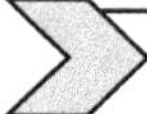 ## 1.6   NABL Accreditation

1.6.1 Introduction

Accreditation is the formal recognition, authorization and registration of a laboratory that has demonstrated its capability, competence and credibility to carry out the tasks it is claiming to be able to do. It provides feedback to laboratories as to whether they are performing their work in accordance with international criteria for technical competence. The concept of laboratory accreditation was developed to provide third-party certification that a laboratory is competent to perform the specific test or type of tests. Laboratory accreditation is a means to improve customer confidence in the test reports issued by the laboratory so that the clinicians and through them the patients shall accept the reports with confidence.

Four years ago, NABL established links with international bodies - Asia Pacific Laboratory Accreditation Cooperation and International Laboratory Accreditation Cooperation. This has imparted international recognition to NABL accredited laboratories. The international standard currently followed by NABL is ISO 15189, specific for medical laboratories

The National Accreditation Board for Testing and Calibration Laboratories (NABL) is an autonomous body under the agencies of the Dept. of Science & Technology, Govt. of India, and is registered under the Societies Act. NABL. Govt. of India has authorized NABL as the sole accreditation body for testing and calibration laboratories.

1.6.2   Objectives

- NABL was initially established with the objective to provide accreditation to testing & calibration laboratories, later on extended its services to the clinical laboratories in our country.

- The objective of NABL is to provide third party assessment of quality and technical competence.

1.6.3   WHY Accreditation

- Accreditation is the third-party attestation related to a conformity assessment body conveying the formal demonstration of its competence to carry out specific conformity assessment task. Conformity Assessment Body (CAB) is a body which includes Testing including medical Laboratory, Calibration Laboratory, Proficiency Testing Provider, Certified Reference Material Producer.

- The liberalization of trade and industry policies of the Government of India has created quality consciousness in domestic trade and provided greater thrust for export. As a consequence, testing centres and laboratories have to demonstrably operate at an internationally acceptable level of competence.

- Laboratory accreditation is a procedure by which an authoritative body gives formal recognition of technical competence for specific tests/ measurements, based on third party assessment and following international standards.

- Similarly, Proficiency testing Provider accreditation gives formal recognition of competence for organizations that provide proficiency testing. Reference Material Producers Accreditation gives formal recognition of competence to carry out the production of reference materials based on third party assessment and following international standards.

1.6.4 Benefits of Accreditation

Formal recognition of competence of a laboratory by an Accreditation body in accordance with international criteria has many advantages.

1. Increased confidence in Testing/ Calibration Reports issued by the laboratory

2. Better control of laboratory operations and feedback to laboratories as to whether they have sound Quality Assurance System and are technically competent

3. Potential increase in business due to enhanced customer confidence and satisfaction.

4. Customers can search and identify the laboratories accredited by NABL for their specific requirements from the NABL Web-site or Directory of Accredited Laboratories

5. Users of accredited laboratories enjoy greater access for their products, in both domestic and international markets.

6. Savings in terms of time and money due to reduction or elimination of the need for re-testing of products.

1.6.5 Scope of Accreditation

NABL Accreditation is currently given in the following fields and disciplines. The multi-disciplinary CABs shall have to apply in relevant discipline separately depending upon to which discipline the scope belongs. For more details on scope of accreditation please refer the relevant specific criteria.

TESTING LABORATORIES	CALIBRATION LABORATORIES	MEDICAL LABORATORIES
• Biological • Chemical • Electrical • Electronics • Fluid-Flow • Mechanical • Non-Destructive Testing (NDT) • Photometry • Radiological Forensic • Diagnostic Radiology QA Testing • Software & IT System	• Electro-Technical • Mechanical • Fluid Flow • Thermal • Optical • Radiological • Medical Devices	• Clinical Biochemistry • Clinical Pathology • Haematology & Immunohematology • Microbiology & Infectious Disease Serology • Histopathology • Cytopathology • Flow Cytometry • Genetics • Nuclear Medicine *(in-vitro tests only)*

MEDICAL IMAGING-CONFORMITY ASSESSMENT BODIES (MI-CAB)

• Projectional Radiography & Fluoroscopy

   a. X-Ray, Bone Densitometry (DEXA), Dental X-Ray-OPG, Mammography etc.

   b. Fluoroscopy

• Computed Tomography (CT)

• Magnetic Resonance Imaging (MRI)

• Ultrasound and Colour Doppler

• Nuclear Medicine

   a. SPECT

   b. PET CT

   c. PET MRI

PROFICIENCY TESTING PROVIDERS	REFERENCE MATERIAL PRODUCERS
• Testing • Calibration • Medical • Inspection	• Chemical Composition • Biological & Clinical Properties • Physical Properties • Engineering Properties • Miscellaneous Properties

1.6.6 Getting Ready for Accreditation

It is very important for a laboratory to make a definite plan for obtaining accreditation and nominate a responsible person as QUALITY MANAGER (who should be familiar with the laboratory's existing quality system) to co-ordinate all activities related to seeking accreditation.

The laboratory should carry out the following important tasks towards getting ready for accreditation:

a. Contact NABL Secretariat with a request for procuring relevant NABL documents (NABL Contact address and the list of NABL documents given in Annexure-3 and 1, respectively).

b. Get fully acquainted with all relevant documents and understand the assessment Procedure and methodology of making an application.

c. Train a person on Quality Management System and Internal Audit (4-day residential training courses conducted by NABL. Contact NABL Secretariat for details).

d. Prepare QUALITY MANUAL as per ISO 15189 standards.

e. Prepare Standard Operating Procedure for each investigation carried out in the laboratory.

f. Ensure effective environmental conditions (temperature, humidity, storage placement, etc.).

g. Ensure calibration of instruments / equipment. Only NABL ACCREDITED CALIBRATION LABORATORIES are authorized to provide calibration. NABL website gives the names of NABL accredited calibration laboratories in the various fields of Accreditation.

h. Impart training on the key elements of documentation, such as document format, authorization of document, issue and withdrawal procedures, document review and change, etc. Each document should have ID No., name of controlling authority, period of retention, etc.

i. Ascertain the status of the existing quality system and technical competence with regard to NABL standards and address the question "Is the system documented and effective OR does it need modification?".

j. Remember Quality Manual is a policy document, which has to be supplemented by a set of other next level documents. Therefore, ensure that these documents are well prepared.

k. Ensure proper implementation of all aspects that have been documented in the Quality Manual and other documents.

l. Incorporate Internal Quality Control (IQC) practice while patients' samples are analysed.

m. Document IQC data as well as uncertainty of measurements. Maintain Levy Jennings charts.

n. Participate in External Quality Assessment Schemes (EQAS). If this is not available for certain analytes, participate in inter-laboratory comparison through exchange of samples with NABL accredited laboratories.

o. Document corrective actions on IQC / EQA outliers.

p. Conduct Internal Audit and Management Review.

q. Apply to NABL along with appropriate fee.

1.6.7 Process of Accreditation

Stage I (Filling of Application)

- Prepare your laboratory's application for NABL accreditation, giving all desired information and enlisting the test(s) / calibration(s) along with range and measurement uncertainty for which the laboratory has the competence to perform. Laboratory can apply either for all or part of their testing / calibration facilities. Formats NABL 151, NABL 152 & NABL 153 are to be used by Testing, Calibration and Medical Laboratories respectively for applying to NABL for accreditation.

- Laboratory has to take special care in filling the scope of accreditation for which the laboratory wishes to apply. In case, the laboratory finds any clause (in part or full) not applicable to the laboratory, it shall furnish the reasons.

- Laboratories are required to submit five sets of duly filled in application forms for each field of testing / calibration along with five sets of Quality Manual and Application Fees.

- NABL Secretariat on receipt of application will issue acknowledgement to the laboratory. After scrutiny of application for it being complete in all respects, a unique Customer Registration Number will be allocated to laboratory for further processing of application.

- NABL Secretariat shall then nominate a Lead Assessor for giving Adequacy Report on the Quality Manual / Application submitted by the laboratory. A copy of Adequacy Report by Lead Assessor will be provided to Laboratory for taking necessary corrective action, if any. The laboratory shall submit Corrective Action Report. After satisfactory corrective action by the laboratory, a Pre-Assessment audit of the laboratory will be organised by NABL. Laboratories must ensure their preparedness by carrying out its internal audit before Pre-Assessment.

Stage II (Pre-Assessment audit)

- NABL Secretariat shall organise the Pre-Assessment audit, which shall normally be carried by Lead Assessor at the laboratory sites.

- The pre-assessment helps the laboratory to be better prepared for the Final Assessment. It also helps the Lead Assessor to assess the preparedness of the laboratory to undergo Final Assessment apart from Technical Assessor(s) and Total Assessment Man-days required vis-à-vis the scope of accreditation as per application submitted by the laboratory.

- A copy of Pre-Assessment Report will be provided to Laboratory for taking necessary corrective action on the concerns raised during audit, if any.

- The laboratory shall submit Corrective Action Report to NABL Secretariat.

- After laboratory confirms the completion of corrective actions, Final Assessment of the laboratory shall be organized by NABL.

Stage III (Final Assessment)

- NABL Secretariat shall organize the Final Assessment at the laboratory site(s) for its compliance to NABL Criteria and for that purpose appoint an assessment team.

- The Assessment Team shall comprise of a Lead Assessor and other Technical Assessor(s) in the relevant fields depending upon the scope to be assessed.

- Assessors shall raise the Non-Conformance(s), if any, and provide it to the laboratory in prescribed format so that it gets the opportunity to close as many Non-Conformance(s) as they can before closing meeting of the Assessment.

- The Lead Assessor will provide a copy of consolidated report of the assessment to the laboratory and send the original copy to NABL Secretariat. Laboratory shall take necessary corrective action on the remaining Non-Conformance(s) / other concerns and shall submit a report to NABL within a maximum period of 2 months.

Stage IV (Corrective Reassessment)

- After satisfactory corrective action by the laboratory, the Accreditation Committee examines the findings of the Assessment Team and recommends additional corrective action, if any, by the laboratory.

- Accreditation Committee determines whether the recommendations in the assessment report is consistent with NABL requirements as well as commensurate with the claims made by the laboratory in its application.

- Laboratory shall have to take corrective action on any concerns raised by the Accreditation Committee.

- Accreditation Committee shall make the appropriate recommendations regarding accreditation of a laboratory to NABL Secretariat.

- Laboratories are free to appeal against the findings of assessment or decision on accreditation by writing to the Director, NABL.

- Whenever possible NABL will depute its own technical personnel to be present at the time of assessment as Coordinator and NABL Observer. Sometimes, NABL may at its own cost depute a newly trained Technical Assessor as "Observer" subject to convenience of the laboratory to be accessed.

Stage V (Granting of Accreditation)

- Accreditation to a laboratory shall be valid for a period of 3 years and NABL shall conduct periodical Surveillance of the laboratory at intervals of one year.

- Laboratory shall apply for Renewal of accreditation to it at least 6 months before the expiry of the validity of accreditation.

UNIT 2

Industrial Organization, Personnel, Equipment and Raw Materials

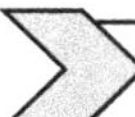

2.1 Organisation and Personnel

Structure of the organization: Organization of the QC department is divided into Quality control- all inspection and testing and Quality assurance- all systems and procedures including batch review and audit. Requirements of US-FDA shall have the responsibility and authority to approve or reject all components adequate laboratory facilities for testing and approval of components

Responsibilities of US-FDA: It has the responsibility for approving or rejecting all procedures or specifications affecting identity, strength, quality, and purity of the drug product. For this written procedure should be followed.

2.1.1 Definition

Quality assurance: Planned and organized activities to help ensure that certain requirements for quality will be met.

Quality control: Operational techniques or tasks that are in place to find and correct problems that may occur.

Functions: Quality must be a prime consideration in the research and Development of a medicine to assure safety and efficacy.

Using a management organization chart (or other tool), the company should illustrate how the quality assurance system fits into the plant organization and how the program's principles, directives and strategies are applied in daily activities.

Quality Manual

The typical contents of a quality manual would contain the following information:

- Quality policy

- General responsibilities
- Sampling procedures
- Equipment testing and release of components
- Reserve samples
- Periodic inspection of stocks, labels and other printed materials
- Vendor selection and
- R and d department stability studies program

Manufacturing Operations and Control

(a) Master Formula Files

(b) Weighing and Dispensing

(c) Processing

(d) In-process Control

(e) Specific Instructions for Sterile Products

(f) Calibration Program g) Validation

(g) Complaints

(h) Returned Goods and their Disposal

(i) Product Recalls

(j) Engineering and Maintenance

(k) Training Program

(l) Audits

Main responsibility of QA and QC Department is to test and control the:

- Ingredient, record, equipment, reagents
- Active pharmaceutical ingredient (API)
- Analytical test report
- Analytical worksheet
- Calibration Certificate of analysis
- Certified reference material
- Compliance testing
- Control sample
- Drug Marketing authorization (product licence, registration certificate)
- Pharmaceutical excipient
- Pharmaceutical product
- Qualification of equipment
- Quality assurance system

- Quality control
- Quality manual
- Reference material
- Reference substance (or standard)
- Secondary reference substance
- Standard operating procedure (SOP)
- Standard uncertainty
- System suitability test
- Validation of an analytical procedure
- Verification of an analytical procedure.
- Verification of performance

2.1.2 Personnel

- To review general issues related to personnel
- To review requirements for key personnel
- To review the training of personnel
- To consider some specific issues Objectives

Principle

Establishment and maintenance of satisfactory system of QA, manufacture and control of products and actives rely on people. There must be sufficient qualified personnel to carry out tasks. Individual responsibilities must be clearly defined and understood by individuals concerned. All personnel should be aware of the principles of GMP that affect them.

2.1.3 General

- Adequate number of persons with necessary qualifications with practical experience are required. An individual's responsibilities should not be so extensive as to present a risk to quality.

- All responsible staff should have specific duties recorded in individual written job descriptions. They should have adequate authority to carry out responsibilities and may delegate to designated deputies with qualifications.

- All personnel should be aware of GMP and must receive training in GMP: -initial training -continuing training -including hygiene standards. They should be motivated to -support the establishment -maintain high-quality standard.

- Prevent unauthorized access -To production areas -Storage areas - Quality control. Stop personnel who do not work in these areas using them as passageways.

Key personnel (which normally should be full-time) positions include

- Authorized persons
  - o Head of Production
  - o Head of Quality Control
- They may delegate functions but not responsibility. Heads of Production and Quality Control should be independent of each other
- These personnel should possess appropriate qualifications and scientific education such as: chemistry or biochemistry, chemical engineering, microbiology, pharmaceutical sciences and technology pharmacology and toxicology physiology; or other related science subjects relevant to the responsibilities to be undertaken.
- They should possess appropriate experience in manufacture and quality assurance.
- Preparatory period under professional guidance sometimes needed which should enable personnel to take difficult decisions in an independent, professional and scientific way to resolve the problems encountered in manufacturing and QC.

2.1.4 Personnel Shared Responsibilities

- Heads of Production and Quality Control may share/jointly exercise some responsibilities relating to quality: authorization of written procedures (SOPs) and other documents, including amendments monitoring and control of manufacturing environment plant hygiene process validation and calibration training, including application and principles of QA approval and monitoring of suppliers and contract acceptors.
- Designation and monitoring of storage conditions for materials and products, Performing and evaluating in-process controls, Retention of records, Monitoring compliance with GMP Inspection, investigation, and taking of samples to monitor factors which may affect quality.

Head of Production: Responsibilities

- Product production and storage according to appropriate documentation
- Approval and implementation of production instructions
- In-process QC and ensure strict implementation
- Ensures that production records are evaluated and signed by designated person

- Checks maintenance of production department, premises and equipment
- Ensures process validation and calibration performed, recorded, and reports are made available
- Ensures initial and continuous training of production personnel

Head of Quality Control: Responsibilities

- Approval or rejection of materials, e.g. packing materials, intermediates, bulk and finished products, in accordance with specifications
- Evaluation of batch records
- Ensures carrying out of necessary testing
- Approval of quality control procedures, e.g. sampling and testing; specifications
- Approval and monitoring of all contract analysis
- Checks maintenance of quality department, premises and equipment
- Ensures validation (including analytical procedure validation) and calibration of control equipment
- Ensures initial and continuous training of QC personnel

Authorized person: Responsibilities

- Compliance with technical and regulatory requirements
- Approval of the release of finished product for sale
- Establishment and implementation of quality system
- Development of quality manual
- Supervision of self-inspections and quality audits
- Oversight of the QC department
- Participation in external audits and vendor audits
- Participation in validation programmes
- May delegate approval of release of product through approved procedure
- Normally by QA by means of batch review

Person releasing the batch should ensure:

- Each batch meets manufacturing and marketing authorization requirements.
- Principles and requirements of GMP are met All checks and tests have been performed.
- Production conditions and manufacturing records.

- Planned changes and deviations reported - including where necessary to drug regulatory authority.

- Additional sampling, inspection, checks and tests had been done when required.

- All production and control documents are completed and endorsed.

- Audits, inspections and spot-checks were done.

- QC approval has been given.

- All other relevant factors have been considered.

2.1.5 Personnel Qualification

Each person engaged in the manufacture, processing, packing, or holding of a drug product shall have education, training, and experience, or any combination thereof, to enable that person to perform the assigned functions. Each person responsible for supervising the manufacture, processing, packing, or holding of drug product shall have the education, training, and experience, or any combination thereof to perform assigned functions in such a manner as to provide assurance that the drug product has the safety, identity, strength, quality, and purity that it purports or is represented to possess. There shall be an adequate number of qualified personnel to perform and supervise the manufacture, processing, packing, or holding of each drug product.

2.1.6 Personnel Responsibilities

- Personnel engaged in the manufacture, processing, packing, or holding of a drug product shall wear clean clothing appropriate for the duties they perform.

- Protective apparel, such as head, face, hand, and arm coverings, shall be worn as necessary to protect drug products from contamination.

- Personnel shall practice good sanitation and health habits.

- Only personnel authorized by supervisory personnel shall enter those areas of the buildings and facilities designated as limited-access areas.

- Any person shown at any time (either by medical examination or by supervisory observation) to have an apparent illness or open lesions that may adversely affect the safety or quality of drug products shall be excluded from direct contact with components, drug product containers, closures, in-process materials, and drug products until the condition is corrected or determined competent medical personnel not to jeopardize the safety or quality of drug products.

Responsibility of Personnel Specialist

- Human resource planning
- Formulation of programmes & procedures
- Employee health & safety programmes
- Training and development of personnel
- Wage & salary administration
- Good labour management relations – grievance handling
- Employee benefit programmes
- Personnel research
- Personnel audit & review work

Functions of Personnel Department

- Formulating policies & procedure
- Manpower Planning Training & Development
- Recruitment & Promotion Service Condition
- Wage & Salary Administration
- PAS & Counselling
- Formulation of various welfare schemes

Training

Under a quality system, managers are expected to establish training programs that include the following:

- Evaluation of training needs
- Provision of training to satisfy these needs
- Evaluation of effectiveness of training
- Documentation of training and/or re-training
- Developing, maintaining, and administering the facility training plan

Training

Training should be in accordance with a written and approved programme of all personnel whose duties take them into production areas; or into control laboratories; and for others whose activities could affect the quality of the product including technical, maintenance and cleaning personnel. Induction and continuing training on theory and practice of GMP should be made mandatory. Their duties training records should be kept practical.

Specific training should be given to staff in special areas, e.g. where contamination is a hazard including clean areas; or areas where highly active, toxic, infectious, sensitizing materials are handled. The concept of

QA should be fully discussed during training to facilitate proper understanding to ensure its implementation.

Visitors or Untrained Personnel

It is preferable not to enter production and control areas. If this is unavoidable then:

- They must be given information in advance, particularly about personal hygiene protective clothing requirements.

- Must be accompanied and closely supervised at all.

2.1.7 Types of Training

1. Initial training programmes for the initial training of newly recruited personnel or personnel taking over new functions should take into account all relevant tasks and procedures, including general topics such as quality assurance, GMP and computerized systems. The training records should identify at least the trainer, all the specified tasks (including the relevant standard operating procedures) and when the training was completed. The records should be signed by both the trainee and the trainer.

2. **Continuous training:** Continuous training programmes (theoretical and/or practical training) should be in place to ensure that personnel keep up the skills to carry out their assigned tasks. Such training programmes should take technical and scientific developments into account. Training should also include any changes to standard operating procedures and personnel requirements. Both internal and external training courses may be useful here.

3. **Competency**: The overall competency of personnel is a result of education, experience and training. As a key factor for the quality and safety of blood and blood products, competency has to be carefully evaluated and continuously monitored. Upon completion of the initial training, the competency of the personnel should be evaluated and documented. After the initial competency is determined, there should be periodic assessment of competency. The contents of training programmes and their effectiveness should be periodically reviewed and assessed.

2.1.8 Personnel Hygiene

- Steps should be taken to ensure as far as is practicable that no person affected by an infectious disease or having open lesions on the exposed surface of the body is engaged in the manufacture of medicinal products. Every person entering the manufacturing areas should wear protective garments appropriate to the operations to be carried out.

- Eating, drinking, chewing or smoking, or the storage of food, drink, smoking materials or personal medication in the production and storage areas should be prohibited. In general, any unhygienic practice within the manufacturing areas or in any other area where the product might be adversely affected should be forbidden. Direct contact should be avoided between the operator's hands and the exposed product as well as with any part of the equipment that comes into contact with the products.

- Personnel should be instructed to use the hand-washing facilities. Any specific requirements for the manufacture of special groups of products, for example sterile preparations, are covered in the annexes.

- Hygiene

- Avoid clean rooms when ill

- Frequent bathing and shampooing

- Avoid getting sunburned

- Avoid cosmetics such as face powder, hair sprays, perfumes and aftershave

- Clothing should be clean, nonfrayed and nonlinting

- Avoid smoking

2.1.9 Personnel Records

Personnel Records are records pertaining to employees of an organization. These records are accumulated, factual and comprehensive information related to concern records and detained. All information with effect to human resources in the organization is kept in a systematic order. Such records are helpful to a manager in various decisions -making areas.

Purposes of Personnel Records

- It helps to supply crucial information to managers regarding the employees.

- To keep an update record of leaves, lockouts, transfers, turnover, etc. of the employees.

- It helps the managers in framing various training and development programmes on the basis of present scenario.

- It helps the government organizations to gather data in respect to rate of turnover, rate of absenteeism and other personnel matters.

- It helps the managers to make salary revisions, allowances and other benefits related to salaries.

- It also helps the researchers to carry in- depth study with respect to industrial relations and goodwill of the firm in the market.

2.1.10 Site Master File

General information:

- Personnel premises and equipment maintenance
- Equipment qualification, validation and calibration
- Sanitation
- Documentation
- Production
- Quality control
- Distribution
- Complaints
- Product
- Recalls
- Self-audit

A Typical Documentation Structure

Quality Manual | Procedures | Work Instructions | Forms | Records

Consultants and contract staff

This regulation is brief and concise regarding the requirements of qualifications for a consultant and what records need to be kept.

Qualifications: Qualification requirements for consultants are the same as those for the facility's employees. The consultant must have the education, training, experience, or a combination of them in the subject or area for which they are advising. If the subject or area involves the drug manufacturing process, then knowledge of GMP regulations is also required. Records: If a company has used a consultant, then a record of this consultant and services provided must be kept. The record must contain, at a minimum, the consultant's name, address, qualifications and type of service provided. Records should prove qualifications. Training records maintained.

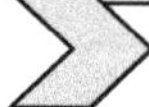 **2.2   Premises**

Content

- Pharmaceutical industry
- Location
- Design & Construction Plan and layout
- Maintenance
- Sanitation

- Environmental
- Control
- Sterile Areas

Pharmaceutical industry

Pharmaceutical industry can be classified arbitrarily on the following:
- Crude and processed botanical drugs
- Fine chemical and pharmaceuticals
- Proprietary drugs

2.2.1 Location

The selection of a location for the construction of a pharmaceutical or chemical plant is a vital decision to be taken, because it determines the balancing of investment and profit. The factory building (s) for manufacture of drugs shall be so situated and shall have such measures as to avoid risk of contamination from external environment including open sewage, drain, public lavatory or any factory which produces disagreeable or obnoxious, odour, fumes, excessive soot, dust, smoke, chemical or biological emissions.

Factors for location
- Fundamental (primary) factors
- Derived (secondary) factors

Fundamental (primary) Factors
- Raw materials
- Market
- Energy availability
- Transportation facility
- Labour supply

Derived (secondary) factors:
- Climate and soil
- Government concession
- Water supply
- Waste disposal
- Site Characteristics
- Flood and Fire Protection
- Community Factors

2.2.2   Design & Construction

The building(s) used for the factory shall be designed, constructed, adapted and maintained to suit the manufacturing operations so as to permit production of drugs under hygienic conditions. They shall conform to the conditions laid down in the Factories Act, 1948 (63 of 1948).

The premises used for manufacturing, processing, warehousing, packaging labelling and testing purposes shall be:

- compatible with other drug manufacturing operations.
- Proper Space for working should be there.
- Proper logically placement of equipment and material
- Avoid the risk of mix-up between different categories of drugs or with raw materials, intermediates and in-process material.
- Control the cross contamination by other drugs or substances.
- Deign should be such that it prevents the entry of insect and rodents.
- Interior surface (walls, floors and ceilings) shall be smooth and free from cracks, and permit easy cleaning, painting and disinfection.
- Provide with adequate lighting and ventilation, if necessary air conditioning to maintain a satisfactory temperature.
- The interior surfaces shall not shed particles.
- A periodical record of cleaning and painting of the premises shall be maintained.
- It should be proper underground drainage system in the processing area as far as possible.
- Sanitary fitting and electrical should be concealed.

Water supply: The water used in manufacture shall be pure and drinkable quality, free from pathogenic microorganism.

Disposal of waste: Waste water and other residues from laboratory which might be prejudicial to worker or the public health shall be disposed of after suitable treatment as per requirement of water pollution control authorities.

2.2.3   Plan and Layout

Plan layout is a coordinated effort to achieve the final objective to integrate machines, material and personal for economic production.

Advantages of plan layout

A proper lay out has the advantages from point of

- Workers

* Labour cost
* Other production cost
* Production controls
* Super- vision
* Capital investment.

Type of plan layout

Plant layouts are of two types:

* Process layout or functional layout
* Product or straight-line layout

2.3.4 Process Layout or Functional Layout

It the arrangement of machines of a particular class doing a particular type of work or process as a separate department. e.g. All cutting machines may be placed in one department. i.e cutting department.

Advantages of process layout:

* More effective supervision can be achieved
* Division of Labour can be provided
* Less disruption occurs in production
* High scope for expansion

Disadvantages: This is not possible in chemical & Pharmaceutical industry.

2.2.4.1 Product or Straight-Line Layout

The arrangement of machines doing various operation in a line as one department. e.g. In manufacture of tablet; dispensing, powder blending, granulation, drying, compression and coating. All of the above look as different operation but logically arranged in a series.

Advantages:

* Process of work will be quick and smooth
* Cost of material handling will be reduced
* Production time is reduced and manufacturing cycle can be speeded up.
* Space of floor can be properly used

2.2.4.2 Factor Influencing Plant Layout

* New site development or additional to developed site.
* Type of Process and product control.
* Space available and space required.

- Operational convenience.
- Economic distribution of utilities and services.
- Health and safety considerations.
- Waste disposal problem.
- Possible future Expansion.

2.2.4.3 Method of Plant and Factory Layout

A proper layout in each case includes arrangement of processing areas, storage area and handling area in efficient co-ordination. The lay out processing units in a plant, the equipment within these units must be planed. Then detail piping, structural and electrical design must be designed. Plan layout play important role in determining construction and manufacture cost.

Different type of information is needed to design an appropriate layout.

- Dimensions of work places.
- Sequence of operations.
- Flow pattern of materials.
- Storage space for raw materials, in process inventory and finished goods.
- Space for offices, aisles, toilets etc

1. **Identification**
2. **Drawings of plant layout**

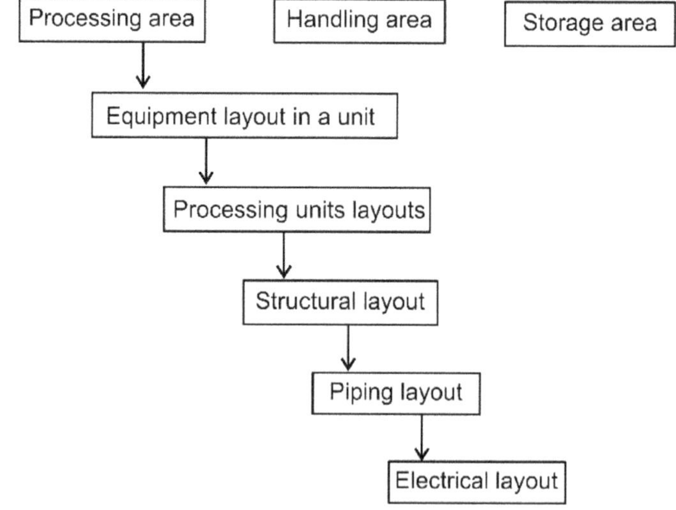

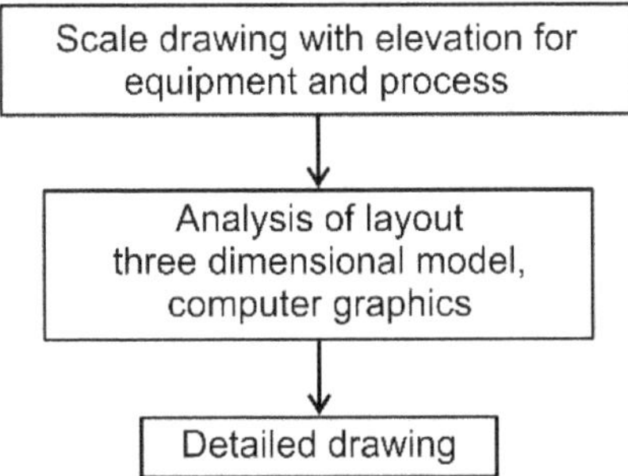

Figure 2.1 Flow diagram of procedures for an appropriate design of plant layout.

2.2.4.4 Special Provision of Pharmaceutical Plant Layout

They shall conform to the condition laid down in Factories Act 1948. The wall of room in which manufacturing operation are carried out shall:

- Have a height of six feet from floor.
- Have smooth and waterproof.
- Be capable of cleaning.
- Flooring shall be smooth, even washable.
- Have no creak and crevices
- Be in such a way as not to permit any retention or accumulation of dust.

2.2.4.5 Raw Material Ware House

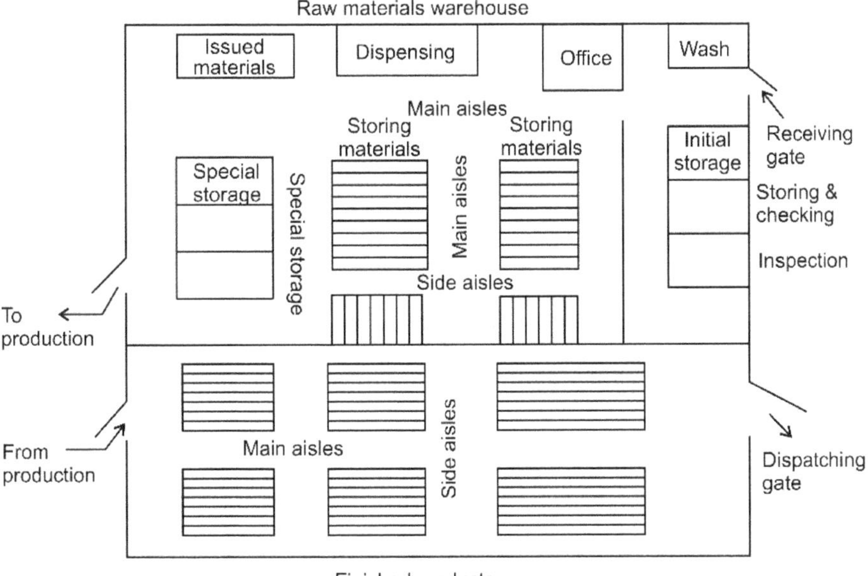

Figure 2.2 Center storage and Perimeter Production.

2.2.5 Maintenance

- Many problems involved in maintenance due to the faculty design and layout of plant and equipment. Sufficient space and facilities for maintenance work must be provided in plant layout. It is essential to consider maintenance regulations while making decisions on equipment.

- Schedule and procedures must be established for the preventive maintenance of equipment. Written procedures must be established for the cleaning and its subsequent release for use in manufacturing.

- Equipments and utensils must be cleaned, stored and wherever appropriate sanitized or sterilized to prevent contamination or carry over.

- Non dedicated equipment must be cleaned between productions of different materials to prevent cross contamination.

2.2.6 Sanitation

- It consists of three things: Sanitary condition; Maintenance Disposal of sewage and Refuse.

- Manufacturing area should not be used for any other purpose. It should be clean, orderly manner and free from accumulated waste, dust, debris etc. Eating, chewing smoking or any unhygienic particle should not permit in manufacturing area. Production areas shall be well lit, particularly where visual on-line controls are carried out.

- A routine sanitation program shall be drawn up and observed, which shall be properly recorded and which shall indicate:
  (a) specific areas to be cleaned and cleaning intervals;
  (b) cleaning procedure to be followed, including equipment and materials to be used for cleaning; and
  (c) personnel assigned to and responsible for the cleaning operation.

2.2.7 Environment Control

- Thermal pollution and control
- Water pollution and control
- Air pollution control

Thermal Pollution and Control

Various off stream cooling system are required to handle thermal discharge from process. There different ways for controlling thermal pollution such as wet cooling towers and dry cooling towers.

Water Pollution

There is a great problem in handling a liquid waste. Liquid effluent is more complex than gas effluent. The treatment could be done by physical treatment, chemical treatment and biological treatment.

Air Control

There are two major categories which are suitable for removing particulate matter. Those associated with removing gaseous pollutant are removal by chemical and physical way.

Sterile Area

For Sterile drugs separate enclosed area specially designed for the purpose shall be provided. Area shall be provided with air locks for entry and shall be essentially dust free and ventilate with air supply. For all areas where aseptic manufacture has to be carried out air supply shall be filtered through HEPA filters and shall be at a pressure higher than in the adjacent area.

Routine microbial counts of all sterile area shall be carried out during manufacturing operation. Area where Manufacturing progress is going on that area must not be occupied by access people. Special procedure should be followed for entering and leaving the manufacturing area

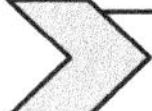 ## 2.3   Equipment

1. Equipment may be defined as a physical entity which is used to carry out a general or specific activity in the pharmaceutical plant. It can be a single piece, for example tablet compression, weighing machine.

2. Equipment is an integrated system that is, group of equipment come together to perform single activity. e.g.: water mineralizing plants, air handling systems.

3. Equipment is generally one of the major inputs along with people facilities, materials, and systems

4. The quality of the manufactured product much depends on the suitability, and level of the technology of the equipment used since it is major requirement in the manufacture of the pharmaceutical products.

5. The regulatory literature on GMP in various countries gives enough importance and provide guide lines on the management of equipment in pharmaceutical plants.

A glance on international GMP literature following points coming up, those are:

- Location and design
- Preventive and breakdown maintenance

- Construction
- Size and adaptation
- Cleaning and cross contamination
- Installation and calibration
- Qualification and validation
- Automatic, mechanical, electronic equipment

2.3.1 Life Stages of Equipment

- Equipment management in the pharmaceutical industry has a life cycle, and the GMP requirement cover the life cycle of equipment.
- It starts with decision to purchase equipment and ends with scrapping or elimination of equipment from operation.
- Decision to purchase equipment is primarily need based.
- It consists of following stages: - decision to purchase equipment - purchase of equipment - qualifying, installing and validating equipment - using the equipment
  1. Availability of spares and servicing.
  2. The frequency and ease of maintenance will significantly impact on productivity and even quality.
  3. Equipment breakdown during processing could adversely affect quality. Included in the maintenance evaluation should be the cleanability of the equipment.
  4. This will involve accessibility to the parts to be cleaned and the relative ease of disassembly and reassembly process.
  5. Environmental issues are important constraints. Is the design of the equipment conductive to the application? Such attributes as the ability to contain toxic products, the ability to maintain aseptic conditions, etc. need to be reviewed.
  6. Construction materials and design.
  7. The type of process controls such as automatic weight adjustment on tablet

Before we take decision to purchase an equipment, we need to look many aspects.

- This primarily helps the user requirement specification for the equipment.
- Following questions may arise in relation to design, size, location, adaption and construction of the equipment.

- Why the need arises for the purchase of equipment e.g. Creation of new facility, increasing capacity, Adapting to new and improved technology
- Which operations we want perform with proposed equipment
- For example, equipment capability analysis, granulation, sterilization.
- What capacity the equipment should have in terms output and holding? E.g. ten lakh tablets per shift or ten thousand litters of liquid.
- How the equipment will be cleaned? And also need to consider that do we face any problem in validating the cleaning process of the equipment?
- Do we have trained operators to operate this equipment? Or whether the manufacturer helps in training our existing operator.
- What will be the starting and stopping time of the equipment?

Following factors are taken into consideration while purchasing the materials:

- Right source
- Right quality
- Right quantity
- Right price
- Right time
- Right mode of transportation

2.3.1.1 WHO Guidelines

- Equipment must be located, designed, constructed, adapted and maintained to suit the operation to be carried out.
- The layout and design of the equipment must aim to minimize the risk of errors and permit effective cleaning and maintenance in order to avoid cross contamination, buildup dust or dirt and in general any adverse effect on the quality of the product.
- Equipment should be installed in such way as to minimize any risk of error or of contamination.
- Production equipment should be designed, located, and maintained to serve its intended purpose.
- Production equipment should be designed, so that it can be easily and thoroughly cleaned on scheduled basis.
- production equipment should not present any hazard to the products.

- The parts of the production equipment that come in to contact with the product must not be reactive, additive or absorptive to an extent that would affect the quality of the product.

- The equipment must be designed to be compatible with most materials and process being used.

2.3.1.2 USFDA Guidelines (211.63)

Equipment used in the manufacturer, processing, packing, or holding of a drug product shall be of appropriate design, adequate size , and suitably located to facilitate operations for its intended use and for its cleaning and maintenance. Equipment shall be constructed so that surface that contact components, inprocess materials, or drug products shall not be reactive, additive, so as to alter the safety, identity, strength, quality or purity of the drug.

2.3.1.3 MHRA/TGA Guide lines

- Any substance required for operation, such as lubricants, shall not come into contact with components drug product containers closures, inprocess materials or drug products.

- So as to alter the safety, identity, strength, quality, purity of the drug product.

- (TGA3.38) equipment should be installed in such a way as to prevent risk of error.

2.3.2 Equipment Identification

- Identification is one of the four quality attributes in the quality of pharmaceutical products.

- The identity of equipment is also important along with the other identifications required just like, product, room, people, system.

- Hence to meet this GMP requirement all equipment must be clearly identified.

2.3.2.1 WHO Guidelines

- Fixed pipe work should be clearly labeled to indicate the contents and were applicable the direction flow.

- All service piping and devices should be adequately marked.

- Special attention paid to the provision of non-interchangeable connections or adaptors for dangerous gases and liquids.

2.3.2.2 US FDA Guidelines

- (211.104): All compounding and storage containers, processing lines, and major equipment used during the production of a batch of a drug product shall be properly identified at all times to indicate their contents.

- (211.105): Major equipment shall be identified by a distinctive identification number or code that shall be recorded in the batch production record to show the specific equipment used in the manufacture of each batch of drug product.

2.3.3   Cleaning and Maintenance

Use of cleaned equipment is one of the basic steps in avoiding contamination and meeting the purity of the product.

2.3.3.1 WHO guidelines

- The layout and design of the equipment must aim to minimize the risk of errors and permit effective cleaning and maintenance in order to avoid cross-contamination build-up of dust or dirt.

- Washing and cleaning equipment should be chosen and used so as to prevent source of contamination.

- Defective equipment should, if possible be removed from production and quality control or at least clearly labeled as defective.

2.3.3.2 MHRA/TGA Guidelines

- (3.35) Repairs and maintenance operations should not present any hazard to the quality of the product.

- Equipment cleaning should be maintained in scheduled bases and that should be recorded in proper way.

2.3.3.3 USFDA Guidelines

- Equipment and utensils shall be cleaned, maintained, and sanitized at appropriate intervals to prevent malfunction or contamination that would alter the safety, identity, strength, purity of the drug product.

- Written procedures shall be established and followed for cleaning and maintenance of equipment.

- A written record of major equipment cleaning, maintenance and use should be included in individual log that show date, time, product, and lot number of each batch processed.

- (21 CFR 211.61) USFDA says that, there should be cleaning SOPs not only for the equipment but also for utensils used in processing.

2.3.3.4 MCC South Africa Guidelines

- A planned preventive maintenance program and sop for carrying out the maintenance should be in place.

- Responsible person should be listed carrying out maintenance in accordance with the specified time schedule.

- Records should be kept as evidence of maintenance checks & repair.

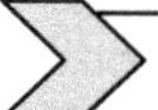

2.4   Raw Materials

All materials that used into the manufacturing of a finished bulk (even though it may not be present in final product e.g. Certain solvents etc.) and which are consumed by person using it are called as raw materials.

Raw materials can be either active drug or inactive substances.

eg. Hard gelatin capsules: even though it is used to fill the blend of medicine, it is not considered as package materials because it is consumed by person using medicines.

2.4.1   Purchase Specification

Definition

Written guidelines that precisely define the operational, physical, and/or chemical characteristics, as well as the quality and quantity of a particular item to be acquired.

2.4.1.1 Mode of Purchasing

- By inspection
- By sample
- By description of brand
- By grading

2.4.1.2 Steps Involved in Purchase Procedure

1. Purchase requisition
2. Selection of supplies
3. Inviting Quotation
4. Placing the order
5. Receiving the material
6. Checking of invoice or bill
7. Recording of bills in books
8. Releasing the payment to the supplier

Staff involved in purchasing have a particular and thorough knowledge of products and suppliers.

- Raw material can be purchased from supplier named in relevant specification or directly from producer.

- Specification established by manufacturer for the starting materials be discussed with suppliers.
- Pharmacist or chemist, who is familiar with quality requirement of various material purchase department can be head of purchase department.

2.4.2   Maintenance of Stores

2.4.2.1 Storage Area Specifications

- Sufficient Capacity
- Clean, dry and maintained within acceptable temperature limit
- Designed and equipped reception area
- Ensuring of quarantine status
- Separate sampling area
- Segregation for storage of rejected, recalled or returned material
- Safe and secure area for narcotics and highly active, dangerous and risky material
- First in First out rule (FIFO)
- First expiring First Out (FEFO)

2.4.2.2 Storage Conditions

- Room temp. Should be $30°$ C and R. H. 60%
- A.C storage ($25\pm 2 °$ C & R.H. $45 - 55\%$)
- Low temp. storage $2 - 8 °$ C
- Separate area for Sterile product storage in A.C
- Light sensitive material in amber color container
- Hermitically sealed container

2.4.2.3 Labelling of Material in Storage Area

- Designated name of product and internal code reference
- Batch no. given by supplier
- Status of Content
- Expiry date or date beyond which retesting is necessary

During fully computerized system used, labelling with all above information need not be necessary.

Check list before storage:

- Integrity of package and seal
- Correspondence notes for the order, delivery and suppliers' labels

Check list during storage

- Separation of rejected, recalled, quarantine, on test, packaging materials.
- Quality of materials

Released by quality control department only.

UNIT 3

Quality Control

When testing is required:

1. New packaging design
2. A revision to current design
3. Change in packaging material

Testing is done before full scale manufacturing to save time and money. Types of test that can be performed or used are:

- Material Testing
- Environmental condition testing (23°C to 50RH)
- Thermal testing (different temperature condition)
- Vacuum testing
- Barrier properties (oxidation, hydrolysis etc. not tested)
- Shock and Impact (Instrument drop)
- Vibrational (while shipping)
- Compression

3.1 Testing of Containers and Closures

3.1.1 Glass Containers for Injectable Preparation

Container intended for injectable preparation maybe ampules, vials or bottles.

Hydrolyic resistance test (IP): 3 types of containers are there;

- Type I
- Type II
- Type III

Type III containers are suitable for use. These types are distinguished by resistance to water attack of new container the degree of attack being determined by amount of alkali release from the glass under the conditions specified:

Normal Capacity of Container (mL)	No. of Containers to be used	Volume of test solution to be used for titration (mL)
5 or less	At least 10	50
6-30	At least 5	50
>30	At least 3	100

Procedure

1. Rinse each container with water at least twice at room temperature.
2. Just before the test rinse each container with freshly prepared distilled water.
3. Determine average overflow volume.
4. Fill container to 90% of their calculated over 1000 volume.
5. Cover with Borosilicate Glass, previously rinsed with freshly prepared distilled water.
6. Place the container in autoclave.
7. Displace the air by passing the steam for 10 minutes.
8. Raise the temperature from 100-120 °C over 20 minutes.
9. Maintain the temperature at 120°C for 69 minutes.
10. Reduce the temperature to 100°C over 40 minutes.
11. Remove the container from autoclave.
12. Cool containers in running water for two minutes.
13. Carryout following titration within 1 hour of removing from autoclave.
14. Combine the liquid from container being examined.
15. Measure the volume of test solution specified in table into a conical flask.
16. Add 0.15 mL of methyl red solution for each 50 mL of liquid.
17. Titrate with 0.01 M HCl.
18. End point colour is obtained by repeating the procedure using the same volume of freshly prepared distilled water.
19. The difference between titration is equal to the volume of 0.01 M HCl required for each 100 mL of test solution.
20. Result should be greater than specified in table.

Capacity of Container (mL)	Volume of 0.01M of HCl /100 mL of test solution Type I or Type II	Type III Glass (1 mL)
<1	2	20
1-2	1.8	17.6
2-5	1.3	13.2
5-10	1	10.2
10-20	0.80	8.1
20-50	0.60	6.1
50-100	0.50	4.8
100-200	0.40	3.9
200-500	0.30	2.9
>500	0.20	2.2

3.1.2 Metal Containers for Eye Ointment

Procedure

1. Select a sample of 50 tubes to be tested
2. Fill the tube with Molten eye ointment base.
3. Close the open ends of each tube through double folds.
4. Allow filled tubes to cool overnight at 15-20°C
5. Assembly a metal bacteriological filter with a paper supported on a perforated plate to a temperature above the melting point for a base.
6. Remove cap from cooled tubes.
7. Apply uniform pressure to the closed ends of each tube in a manner so that the time taken to express as much as possible through each nozzle is 20 seconds.
8. Collect extracted base from each tube.
9. Apply suction to stem of filter when all melted mass has been removed.
10. Wash the walls of filter.
11. Expose the filter paper to 3 successive quantities each of 30 mL $CHCl_3$.
12. Allow filter paper to dry.
13. Examine the filter paper under light with the aid of magnifying glass of 1 mm sq. area.

Note:

- No. of metal particles 1mm in length: 50
- No. in the range of 0.5 to 1mm: 10
- No. in the range of 0.5 to 0.2 mm: 2
- No in the range less than 0.2 mm: Nil

Tube passes the test if total score is low than 100 test tubes. Tubes does not pass the test if score is more than 150, then the test is repeated.

3.1.3 Plastic Containers

1. Testing of Thermoplastic
    (a) Flexural Test: It is among the most common classic method for semi rigid or rigid plastics.
    (b) Pendulum Impact Test: This test is used to measure the behavior of materials at high deformation speeds. Pendulum impact test is used to determine the energy required to break a standardized specimen by measuring the height to which the pendulum hammer rises after impacting the test pieces.
2. Clarity of aqueous test for Oral Liquids

Procedure

1. Select unlabeled, unmarked and non laminated portions from suitable container.
2. Cut this portion into strips. None of which should have total area greater than 20cm square.
3. Wash the strips by shaking them with at least a portion of distilled water for about 30 seconds.
4. Drain of the water
5. Select the wash portions of sample with a total surface area of 125 cm square.
6. Transfer to a flask previously cleaned with chronic acid mixture and rinse with several portions of distilled water.
7. Add 250 mL of distilled water.
8. Cover the flask and autoclave at 121°C for 30 minutes.
9. Carryout blank determination using 250 mL of distilled water.
10. Cool and examine the extract. It should be colourless and free from turbidity.

3.1.4 Test for Rubbers (Closures)

(a) Fragmentation Test:
    1. Place a volume of water in 12 Clean vials. Close vials with closures and **screw** caps for 16 hours **pierce** the closures with 21 SWG. Hypodermic needle (by angle of 10 to 14°) and inject 1 mL water and remove some quantity of air. Repeat the above operation for 4 times for each closure (use new needle for each closure).
    2. Count the no. fragments visible to naked eyes.

3. Total no. of fragments should not be more than 10 expect butyl rubber where the fragments should not exceed 15.

(b) Self Stability Test:

1. Fill 10 vials with water and close the vials with closures.

2. **Pierce** the cap 10 times at different sites with 21 SWG- Hypodermic needle.

3. Immerse the vial in 0.1% w/v solution of methyl blue under reduced external pressure for 10 minutes.

4. Restore the normal pressure and keep the container immersed for 30 minutes.

5. Wash the vial. Name of the vial should contain the trace of colour solution.

3.1.5 Test for Containers

(a) Leakage test:

1. Fill 10 containers with water.

2. Fit closures

3. Keep inverted at room temperature for 24 hours.

4. There should be no sign of leakage from any container.

(b) Collapsibility test for Collapsible tube: A container by collapsing inwards during use should yield at least 90% of its content at required rate of flow.

(c) Transparency test:

1. Standard suspension = 1 g of hydrazine sulphate + sufficient water to produce 100 mL set aside for 6 hours.

2. 25 mL of above solution + 25 mL of w/v hexamine.

3. Mix and allow to stand for 24 hours.

4. 15 mL – dilute to 100 mL.

5. Standard suspension preparation: A 16-fold dilution of standard suspension so as to give an absorbance about 640 nm of 0.37-0.43. Fill the 5 containers with dilute suspension.

6. Compare the cloudiness with container of same type filled with water.

(d) Water Vapour Permeability:

1. Fill 5 containers with water.

2. Heat, seal the bottle with aluminum foil (polyethylene laminate)

3. Weigh accurately each container.

4. Allow to stand for 14 days at RH of 60%+5% and temperature below 20-25°C.
5. Reweigh the container.
6. Loss in weight in each container should not be more than 0.2%.

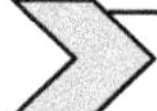 ## 3.2   Good Laboratory Practices (GLP)

GLP are guidelines for the quality control and quality assurance for any work performed by testing laboratories. It can be defined as "GLP is a set of principles that provide a framework following which laboratory studies are planned, performed, monitored, recorded, reported and achieved."

According to WHO, "The GLP regulations set out the rules for good practice and help researchers perform their work in compliance with their own pre-established plans and standardized procedures".

The aim of the GLP regulations is to encourage scientists to organize and perform their studies in a way which promotes the quality and validity of the test data. It also makes the results reliable, repeatable, auditable and recognized worldwide. GLP specifically refers to the quality system of management control for research laboratories or organizations to try to ensure the uniformity, consistency, reliability, reproducibility, quality, integrity of chemical.

3.2.1   Objectives of GLP

The regulations are not concerned with the scientific or technical content of the research programs. Nor do they aim to evaluate the scientific value of the studies. All GLP texts, irrespective of their origin, stress the importance on the following points five points:

1. **Resources:** organization, personnel, facilities and equipment
2. **Characterization:** test items and test systems
3. **Rules:** study plans (or protocols) and written procedures
4. **Results:** raw data, final report and archives
5. **Quality Assurance**

The training program of the WHO covers each of these five fundamental points and explains the requirements of GLP in each case. The major points are summarized below:

3.2.2   Organization and Personnel

GLP regulations require that the structure of R&D organizations and the responsibilities of R&D personnel be clearly defined. GLP also stresses that there should be sufficient staff to perform the tasks required. The qualifications and the training of staff must also be defined and documented. Facilities and equipment. The regulations emphasize the need for sufficient facilities and equipment to perform the studies. All equipment must be in working order. To ensure this, a strict program of qualification, calibration and maintenance must be adopted.

Characterization

In order to perform a study correctly, it is essential to know as much as possible about the materials used during the study. For studies that evaluate the properties of pharmaceutical compounds during non-clinical studies, it is a prerequisite to have details about the test item and the test system (often an animal or plant) to which the test item is to be administered.

Appropriate Technical/Professional Qualification:

WHO guidelines on GLP gives some guideline on the qualification. It states that education should include study of an appropriate combination of:

1. Chemistry (Analytical, organic and Bio-chemistry)
2. Chemical Engineering
3. Microbiological
4. Pharmaceutical Sciences and Technology
5. Pharmacology and Toxicology
6. Other related sciences

In pharma production one should be B. Pharm, M. Pharm, PHD, B.sc Technology, M.sc Technology.

1. **Training of Employee's**

   A person is called trained person when he/she has appropriate knowledge, Skill & Attitude. Here Knowledge refers to the theoretical background expert in a person regarding the job when he/she is going to perform & also the knowledge about the principle of GLP which may affect this area of work.

   Skill refers to the practical experience he has or in other words their ability to use their theoretical knowledge to perform their particular task.

   Attitude it is a behaviour trade of a person who is performing a task they must have knowledge, skill and positive attitudes towards performing works assign to them. Trained Person is one who have knowledge of his job& GLP, Skills.

2. **Sufficient No. of Peoples**

   The manufacturer should have an adequate number of personnel with the necessary qualification and practical experience the responsibilities placed on any one individual should not be so extensive as to present any risk to quality. The sufficiency is to be designed based on the work load. How many plants being operated has direct relevance to the No. of people required.

3. **Ability to perform given task at given level**

4. **People must be trained all the level to perform the designated jobs.**

   - Top Manager and Directors
   - Junior and Senior Manager
   - Floor Supervisors
   - Machine operator

3.2.3 Facilities

It has been stated in general that the testing facility shall be of suitable size, construction and location to facilitate the proper conduct of nom-clinical laboratory studies. It shall be designated so that there the degree of separation that will prevent any function or activity from having any adverse effect on the study.

3.2.3.1 Design and Construction Features

1. Laboratory should be located in area sufficiently free from noise and vibrations to prevent inference with its functions.

2. Sufficient Space to diff. sections of lab to avoid mix-up and cross contamination.

3. Sufficient space for storage.

4. Separate space for locker, shower & washing and sterilization of medicines, glassware's and equipment.

5. Sewage treatment installation.

6. Lab should be well ventilated, free from dust, drafts and extreme temperature.

7. A minimum of 150 sq. feet of floor space should be provided for each analysis.

8. A minimum 6 linear feet of washable bench, space, free of equipment should be provided for each analysis.

9. Separate space should be provided for sensitive instruments.

10. Separate air handling limit should be provided for testing of Bio-Hazardous materials.

11. Both Hot/Cold running water supply.

3.2.3.2 Animal Care Facilities

Many tests require use of animal's laboratories which wish to undertake tests. Requiring different animals should provide animal care facilities. Some guideline which will be useful in designing & construction are given below:

1. Animal care facility should be located away from testing lab, preferably in a separate building.

2. This building should have self-contained ventilation system and should have at least the following segregated areas:

   - Quarantine area foe incanting animals.
   - Area for sick animals.
   - Area for storage of food.
   - Animal incubation area.
   - Animal post-mortem area.
   - Cage dis-infection area, in case of small animals.
   - Waste or dead animal disposal area.
   - Waste and Dead animal disposal area.
   - Shower and changing facilities for staff.

3.2.4 Equipment

- Equipment design
- Maintenance and calibration of equipment
  - **Equipment design:** A variety of equipment are used in a testing laboratory the design may be simple or complex but it should serve intended purpose. Some guidelines which may be useful in relation to equipment are given below:

Laboratory, Glassware, Plasticware and metal utensils

1. Except for disposable plastic ware, these should be resistant to effect of corrosion, high temp. and vigorous learning operation.

2. Plastic item should be of clear inert, non-toxic material and should retain accurate graduation or calibration weak mark.

3. All glassware should be free of chips and cracks.

4. Metal utensils made of stainless steel should be preferred.

5. Culture tube should be of borosilicate glass or other corrosion resistant glass.

6. Dilution bottle should be of borosilicate glass.

Major Instrument

The requirement for instruments depends upon the types of samples that are to be tested in a testing lab. Approved drug testing lab carry out testing of a variety of samples major. e.g. That testing lab requires are:

Analytical Balances, IR Spectrophotometer, U.V, Gas Chromatography, Polarimeter, PH Meter, Disintegration Test Apparatus, Isolation Test Apparatus, Potentiometer, Karl Fisher Titrometer, HPLC, HPTLC.

Equipment for microbiological lab: Autoclave, Microscope, Incubator, Centrifuge Membrane Filter, Colony Counter, Laminar Flow, Hot Air Sterilizer, Refrigeration, Deep Freezer, pH Meter etc.

Maintenance and calibration of equipment: - Lab should prepare program for instrument calibration and preventing maintenance. Objective of the program is to ensure that instruments and equipment need allowable, tolerance and operating properties.

There are three absolute requirements

- Qualified personnel
- Detail Procedure
- Personnel connected with this program should have appropriate qualification and training may include of site seminar on job training
- They should be general description of program or standard operating problem
- SOP should describe the overall objective of the program as the following:
  - (a) The instruments
  - (b) Calibration standards and limits
  - (c) Calibration for each limit
  - (d) Record keeping requirements and logs
  - (e) Instrument's calibration stickering
  - (f) Removals from service of equipment that fails to meet requirements.

There are two broad types of laboratory instruments to be calibrated

(a) One those whose calibration is absolute. eg: measurement of types time.

(b) Those whose calibration is related to a specific standard. eg: pH.

3.2.5 Testing Facilities of Operations

3.2.5.1 SOP

- The testing facilities should have SOP in writing.
- All deviation in studies from SOP should be authorized by the director.

- Significant changes in the established sop shall be properly authorized in writing by management.
- Laboratory manuals and sops should be available immediately to the laboratory area to which they belong.
- A historical fall of all SOPs and all the revision should be maintained

Definition: It can be defined as the written documents specifying the procedure that must be follow to carry out operations.

Purpose of SOP's:

1. To reduce the introduction of error and variation in operation.
2. Historical prospective that is how an operation will be carried out.

How SOP's are Beneficial to Organization

Since SOP's outline the critical aspects of procedure they help to ensure that these aspects are appropriately emphasized. While having out of the procedure.

Individual need to rely on memory or word of mouth communication procedure and this helps to prevent introduction of errors & variation.

It can be used to trained the personnel under training can clarify the aspect which has not clearly understood by them. This helps to prevent misunderstanding.

Preparing an SOP will require an individual to think the whole operation and procedure to be described in doing this. He can identify the potential problems and their solution. This SOP's improve planning and organization.

SOP's eliminate need to developed the procedure every time an operation performed.

Guidelines for Preparation of SOP's

1. Give a clear and descripted tittle to each SOP.
2. Provide sufficient details the SOP must meet the need of an individual, on some time it should be general enough for more than one user.
3. Flexibility should be written in SOP whenever appropriate but it should not be made too general for, it may be use in meeting its intended purpose.
4. Organized SOP according to order of sequence of events involved in performing the operation write the test in straight forward and easy to follow manner.
5. After drafting the SOP used it to perform the operation. To ensure that it has sufficient details and it clear to perform the operation.

6. Take it into account the instruction from manufacturer of the equipment which is employed in performing the operator while drafting the SOP's.

7. Indicate total number of pages so that the user is certain that his performing the complete operation.

8. Indicate the effective date of SOP.

3.2.6   Reagents and Solution

- In the test and analysis reagents and solutions are of critical importance reagents and chemicals should be purchased from reupdated manufacturer.

- Approval of vender could be through a vender certification program.

- It could be ideal if chemicals could be tested for identification test when they are received.

- All the chemicals and reagents are also important reagents which are required to be stored at low temperature. If stored at room temperature May cause their efficacy. When reagents are stored in refrigerator then temperature should be monitored.

- Highly toxic chemical should be stored in appropriate condition in the custody of a responsible person.

3.2.6.1 Reference Materials or Reference Standards

- With the growing use of spectrophotometer, Chromatographic techniques, use of reference standards has grown up.

- Reference standard has high purity and critical characteristics usually reference standard are maintained and distributed by national laboratories and centre designated by National government.

- In India, this responsibility rest with the CDL but due to several factors CDL has been not able to maintain and distribute all the reference standard that are needed by the various drug laboratories.

- To the over this situation the Govt. of India constituted a Committee with the director of CDL as the chairman and the committee has identify 143 items of reference standard.

3.2.7   Test and Control Article

3.2.7.1 Test and Control Article Characterization

(i) In the laboratories attached to the manufacturing unit or in approved drug testing laboratories, control articles may be required only when bioequivalence study are to be made, otherwise the sample received will be test article only.

(ii) The objective of guidelines in this part is to completely define the test article or control article in case of marketed product as control article. It will be characterized by the labelling.

(iii) In contest with testing laboratories attached to the manufacturing unit, a sample collected by quality control personnel should be labelled with the following precautions: -

    (a) Name of the item

    (b) Strength and composition

    (c) Specifications like IP, BP, USP.

    (d) Batch and Lot No.

    (e) Stage at which sample taken

    (f) Name of person who collected Sample

    (g) Date of collection of samples

    (h) Special storage of sample

(iv) In a case sample is received in approved testing laboratories, the laboratory must insist that sample should be labelled with the following particulars: -

    (a) Name of item

    (b) Strength and composition

    (c) Specifications like IP, BP, USP

    (d) Formula in case of patient

    (e) Proprietary Products

    (f) Batch and Lot no.

    (g) Batch Size

    (h) Name of manufactures together with manufacturing lisence no.

    (i) Date of Manufacture and date of date of expiry

    (j) Name of person if other than manufacture submits the sample

    (k) Date of submission of sample

    (l) Quantity of Sample

    (m) Special storage conditions If any

3.2.7.2 Test and Control Article Handling

1. Procedures to be established for handling of test and control articles.

2. One person can be assigned a duty of receiving sample having knowledge about storage conditions of drug. This person can assign a code or other no like job cards no for further handling of sample.

3. A sample should be in appropriate storage conditions while handling the sample when it is distributed through the established procedure to an analyst care should be taken that it is not damaged or contaminated.

4. It should also be ensured that identified is maintained throughout distribution chamber.

5. It has been also be provided that stability of each test or control article should be determined by testing facility.

6. The drug and cosmetics rules provide for retaining reference sample for finished products.

7. WHO, GLP provide for retaining reference samples of both raw material and finished products.

8. Spirit of this concept is to retain reference sample of all test articles so that contra version of result in future can be verified.

9. If it is recommended that laboratories attached with manufacturing units should take up stability studies of each finished products and determine re-test date of each raw material.

3.2.7.3 Protocols for Conducting of Non-clinical Laboratory Studies

Protocol: For writing protocol, a detailed guideline has been given in the tests and readers must refer to them. In India, these guidelines may be referred while preparing test methods for raw material and finished products.

Conduct of Non-Clinical Laboratory Studies

1. These guidelines prescribed that the study shall be conducted in accordance with the protocol and test system shall be monitored.

2. Besides these guidelines for identification of specimens record of gross findings and data entry into the computer have been prescribed.

3.2.8   Records and Reports

3.2.8.1 Reporting of Non-Clinical Laboratory Study Results

1. GLP of US-FDA requires that a final report should be prepared for each non-clinical lab study.

2. This report should be signed by the study director.

3. This amendment should be clearly identifying that part of the final report that is being added to a corrected and addition. This should be signed and dated by the Personnel Responsible.

4. Reporting of result is important element of GLP.

5. Drugs and Cosmetics requires that particular laid down under the **Schedule-U** Should be shown in Analytical Records.

3.2.8.2 Storage and Retrieval of Records and Data

1. GLP of US-FDA provides that these should be archived for orderly storage of all the raw data documentation Protocol. Specimens and final reports and the conditions in the archived should be such that storage would not allow Deterioration of specimen, documents.

2. The provision of contract with commercially achieved has also been provided besides these guidelines some specific requirements are:

   - An individual should be identified as responsible for the archived.

   - Only authorized person should be allowed to enter the archived.

   - Material retained should be index by the test articles, Data of Study test system and Nature of Study.

3.2.8.3 Retention of Records

- Under these guidelines, Specific time periods have been précised for different records, the reader may go through the text.

- In India, Retention Period for Records in respect of drug manufacturer and approved drug laboratory are as under a manufacturer 2 years beyond, the Date of Expiry of each product and 5 years where Date of Expiry were not mentioned.

- Approved Testing Laboratory 2 years beyond the date of expiry of the product and 6 years where Date of Expiry has not been Mentioned.

3.2.8.4 Disqualification of Testing Facilities

- These are the regulatory Provisions and are not relevant to India.

- In India, if a manufacturer is found not complying with the provision of drug and cosmetics act and rules made their under either in respect of manufacturer or testing or both.

- Licensing authority under the said rules can suspend or cancel the license of the manufacturer. However, before doing that licensing authority is required to give the manufacturer a notice in writing of such actions.

- Explanation reasoning is to be heard before such action is taken.

- Similarly, in case of approved drugs testing lab approval can be suspended or cancelled if the laboratory is found not complying with the provisions related to approval.

- Visons related to approval. A similar procedure is to be followed in case of approved testing laboratory.

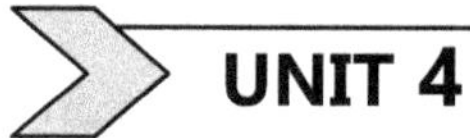 UNIT 4

Complaint

Statement that is something wrong or not good enough, which shows customer dissatisfaction about the company and the product. Example: Complaint about packaging materials, Concerning about the product etc.

Reasons

- It gives the company an opportunity to improve the quality of the product.
- It is helpful to maintain cGMP.
- It maintains committed relationship between the customer and company.
- It is the regulatory obligation.
- Aid in implementing solutions to these quality problems.
- Reduce costs and improve production schedules.
- Reduce employee confusion.
- Improve the safety and performance of device.
- Identify poor performance in the overall quality system, particularly faulty design of devices, and faulty manufacturing processes.
- Verify confidence in, and improve the performance of the quality system.
- Reduce medical device reporting.
- Improve customer relations by reducing the frequency of problems, complaints, and recalls; and,
- Assure compliance with device regulations and consensus standards.

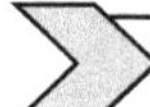 ## 4.1 Types of Complaint

Quality complaints: Originate at consumer level and concern with physical, chemical and biological properties or condition of labeling and /or packaging of the product.

Adverse reaction complaints: Due to allergic reactions of any other untoward reaction or fatal reaction or near fatal reaction.

Other medically related complaints: Include complaints such as lack of efficacy or clinical response.

4.1.1 Steps Involved in Handling of Complaints

Step 1: Receiving Complaints. It is important to have open channels with customers in order to receive their suggestions, doubts and complaints. Generally, these channels are toll-free numbers, e-mails, chat-rooms and P.O. boxes. Whatever the channel, it is necessary to have a person in charge of receiving the complaints and in putting them into an appropriate investigation form that shall be addressed to the Quality Assurance (QA) unit for investigation.

Step 2: Technical Investigation. Upon receipt of the investigation form, the QA unit is able to start the investigation, which can be divided in two phases:

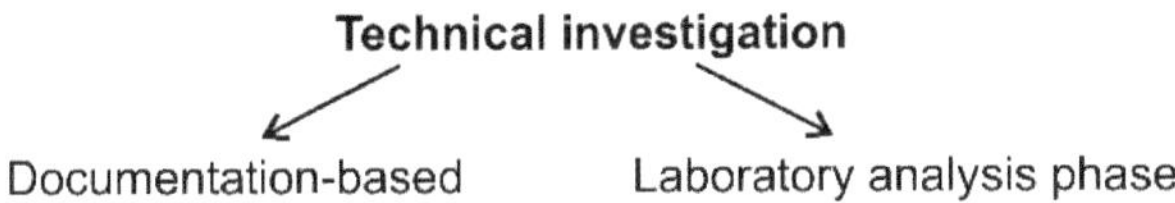

Documentation-based: Checking if this complaint occurred previously in the same lot or if any nonconformance was found in the lot during its production.

1. **Laboratory analysis phase:** Requesting QC laboratory to analyze both samples (complaint & retained). If the customer did not send the complaint sample for analysis, the lab. Investigation will be carried out only with the retained.

2. **Non-confirmed complaint:** When both complaint and retained samples showed results in compliance with specifications or when only the complaint sample showed OOS results that cannot be considered a single unexplained failing product. OOS results in a complaint sample can be attributed to misuse or mishandling.

   Example: Tablets of the complaint sample show a change in their appearance that is characteristic of a light, humidity or high temperature exposure.

3. **Counterfeit / tamper suspicion:** When the retained sample is within the specification but the complaint sample is clearly OOS with no reason for that, such as a counterfeit or tampered drug product.

   Example: When packaging material is different from the original; an example of tampering is when the color of the drug product is completely different from the original or when any foreign substance was added to the product.

Step 3: Corrective Actions and Feedback to Customers: Corrective actions can range from a simple and quick training to some employees to a formal Corrective Action and Preventive Action (CAPA) handling. The criteria for choosing appropriate action depend on the nature of the complaint, and the complaint incidence. If a CAPA is opened, a multidisciplinary team consisting of representatives of QA, QC, Regulatory Affairs and Production Management must be established.

As feedback to the customer, the company must write a response letter to the complainant to explain the investigation approach taken, the results obtained and any implications, in case the quality problem was confirmed.

The customer should be sent a free replacement product together with the response letter, since the customer returned the product (the "complaint sample") to the company for analysis and a quality problem was found.

Concerning non-confirmed complaints originating from misuse or inadequate handling of the drug product, even if there is no need for internal corrective actions, corrective measures should be implemented to provide orientation to the customer.

Step 4: Monthly Reports and Trend Analysis

Monthly reports should be elaborated in order to evaluate the amount and the nature of the complaints received and to perform a trend analysis of these complaints. The monthly reports must answer the following questions:

- How many complaints did the company receive in the period?
- How many were confirmed?
- How many were non-confirmed or were counterfeit/tamper suspicion?

4.1.2 Product Complaint Data Sheet

- Serial number assigned to the complaints.
- Exact nature of the complaints.
- Name of the complainants.
- Address of the complainants.
- Date of complaint received.
- If verbal, name of the person who received the complaint.
- Name of the product, strength and batch number of the product.
- Reference to analytical record number
- Quantity involved in the complaint.

- Size of sample obtained from the complainant.
- Evaluation of complaint by QC department.
- Materials and records used to perform evaluation.
- Other possible effected materials, products and results of their investigation.
- Name and signature of the investigator(s) and date.
- Action taken by the company.
- Copy of reply sent to complainant.

4.1.3 Complaint Record

Name and address of complainant;

- Name (and, where appropriate, title) and phone number of person submitting the complaint;
- Complaint nature (including name and batch number of the bulk product or Medicinal Product/Drug);
- Date complaint is received;
- Action initially taken (including dates and identity of person taking the action);
- Any follow-up action taken;
- Response provided to the originator of complaint (including date response sent); and
- Final decision on bulk product or Medicinal Product/Drug batch or lot.

Customer Complaint Record Book

Report no	Date received	Product name	Received by Product	Lot number	Date investigation started	Date investigation ended

1. **Objective:** To lay out the procedure for investigation and reporting the market complaints.
2. **Responsibility:** The quality assurance manager along with manager of the complaint related department.
3. **Accountability:** The Head, Q.A / Q.C / Regulatory shall review the investigation report, suggest corrective actions and approve the complaint report.

4. Procedure:

1. Market complaint may be received from any of the following sources: Physicians, Pharmacist, Warehouse, Patients, Regional Offices, Hospitals Regulatory affairs, Wholesale Traders, Actual users.

2. Complaints shall be classified in following categories to facilitate investigation: Product quality complaints (non-therapeutic). - Packaging complaints (shortages and packaging error). - Medical complaints (therapeutic problems).

3. As a company policy even, verbal complaints shall be formalized and investigated.

4. All written and oral complaints to be forwarded to Head, QA/QC/Regulatory or his nominee for investigation.

5. All the Product Quality Complaints shall be investigated jointly with QA/F and D/Manufacturing within 5 days of the receipt of the complaint.

6. Medical complaint investigations shall be carried out jointly by Medical department, QA, Production, F and D and Marketing Department within 3 days of receipt of complaint.

7. Packaging complaints and Quality complaints shall be jointly investigated by QA, F and D and Manufacturing department within 10 days of receipt of complaint.

8. The investigator shall investigate the complaint by referring to the Batch Manufacturing Record, SOP, machine log tables, retain samples, reconciliation of materials, storage conditions used and prepare the Product Complaint Report (PCR).

9. The PCR (Annexure I) shall include the product details, details of the complainant, quantity involved, enclosed complaint sample (if any), details of investigation actions taken and recommended corrective actions to prevent such recurrences in future. Each PCR shall be approved by Head/QA/QC/Regulatory or his nominee.

10. Incase of the Head/QA/QC/Regulatory finds that investigation is not necessary, such written records shall be maintained including reasons for not conducting the investigation.

11. Each report shall be assigned a specific PCR number, which will be a 3-digit number starting with "001" in continuous sequence prefixed with "PCR" and suffixed with the last two digits of the year. For example, the first market complaint for 2006 shall have the number PCR/001/006.

12. If product defect is established or suspended in a batch, Head/QA/QC/Regulatory will decide for checking other batches in order to determine whether they are also affected.

13. In case of medical complaints, if Head, /QA /QC /Regulatory and Medical Advisor feels that the product will put the public at risk, he shall advise immediate recall of the batch. The depth of recall is dependent on the seriousness of the complaint.

14. Complaint Record shall be maintained at least one year after expiration date of medicine.

15. Complaint Record shall be reviewed and a monthly summary shall be prepared for the management.

16. A Register is maintained having the complete details of complaint for future reference.

ANNEXURE – 1

PRODUCT COMPLAINT REPORT

Product Name:			Complaint Category: Packaging / Quality / Medical
Batch no.	Mfg. Date	Expiry Date	Packaging Details:
Name / Address Of Complainant:			Reference No. / Date
Complaint Reported Through:			Reference No. / Date
Complaint Sample Enclosed: Yes / No Quantity Of Sample Enclosed:			Total Quantity Involved
Details Of Product Complaint:			
Investigation Report (Additional Sheets To Be Attached If Necessary)			PCR Received By On : Investigation Done By :
Action Taken			Conclusion : Confirmed / Not Confirmed PCR No. : PCR Approved By :
Recommended Corrective Actions			

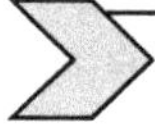

4.2   Handling of Return Goods (Drug Product / Material)

Returned Goods:

- The material which fails to meet the established specification, at the customer's end or the material which does not meet the customer's specification.

- The material, which has been returned on the basis of breakage / damaged packaging, commercial or administrative aspects, or on the basis of customer complaint Investigation and action thereof.

- Withdrawal of specific batch/batches from the market, based on product recall procedure.

Re-Dressing:

- It is defined as repacking of the drug substance without disturbing its original inner bag (Primary packing material) by only changing its label or outer drum (secondary packing material) for commercial purpose.

4.2.1 Purpose

- The purpose of this SOP is to define the procedure for handling, redressing, and repacking of finished goods/ returned goods.

4.2.2 Scope

- This procedure is applicable for handling, redressing, and repacking of finished goods due to revised price, shelf-life extension, (conversion of sale pack to physician's sample pack or vice versa) and returned goods, returned from any other location/Market.

4.2.3 Responsibilities – Handling of Returned Goods

- Warehouse (BSR) personnel shall inform to quality assurance & production department about the receipt of returned finished goods and maintain the records of returned goods.

- Warehouse (BSR) personnel shall check all the documents and conditions of return goods and shall store the returned goods as per the recommended condition.

- Quality Assurance personnel shall verify the physical condition of return goods and ensure that the laydown procedure is followed as per SOP.

- QA personnel shall provide BPR in case of Redressing/Repacking of finished goods/ returned goods and shall withdraw the control sample, and release the batch after the completion of all packing activities.

- Quality Control personnel shall analyze returned goods as per recommendation by QA Head.
- Production personnel shall plan for packing as per the action suggested by QA Head and shall generate BOM, work order, and MRO as per the requirement.
- The plant Head and Quality Head shall be responsible for the review and approval of the SOP and to ensure the compliance of this laydown procedure.

4.2.4   Abbreviations – Handling of Returned Goods

- **BOM:** Bill of Material
- BSR: Bonded Store Room
- BPR: Batch Packing Record
- COA: Certificate of Analysis
- GIM: Goods Inward Memo

4.2.5   Procedure – Handling of Returned Goods

Receipt and handling of returned goods:

- Warehouse (BSR) personnel shall receive the returned goods from the market or any other location.
- Store the materials on separate pallets as per the appropriate storage condition of the respective products in the designated area of return goods or in the other area by identifying with blue rope/net (if space is not available in the designated area).
- **After receipt of the material, the warehouse shall verify the returned consignment for the following points against receipt documents received.**
    - Identity of the product / authenticity of labels.
    - Batch Number
    - The number of containers/shippers received against supply.
    - Condition of containers/shipper's intactness and seal integrity.
    - Weight and the total quantity of returned goods containers/ shippers.
    - Warehouse personnel shall check the physical condition of returned goods and record the details in the "Returned Goods Verification Report".
    - Warehouse personnel shall generate "Distribution Receipt" and prepare a GIM in the system on the basis of originally

acknowledged challan, and confirm the system generated "Goods Returned Settlement Memo".

- In case of any discrepancy in the receipt documents, warehouse shall not confirm the "Goods Returned Settlement Memo" and intimate to concern person/ customer/ marketing department/ other location, for its rectification.

- After rectification of discrepancy in receipt documents warehouse shall confirm the "Goods Returned Settlement Memo" in the system.

- After the generation of "Distribution Receipt" in the system and physical verification of returned goods,

- Warehouse personnel shall send the "Returned Goods Verification Report", to the QA for verification.

- **QA shall verify the goods consignment and shall recommend for decision-based on the following:**
  - If, the material is returned due to commercial dispute or due to not meeting with physical parameters;

  - In case if the material is found intact, the seal number and label number are matching with packing details, then the decision shall be taken by management to release the material for re-sale directly.

  - If, the material is returned from the customer on the commercial dispute or due to not meeting with physical parameters, or the seal is broken by the customer,

  - QA shall verify the material and based on observation.

  - If the material is found to be contaminated or if it is the case of sabotage, the same shall be sent for destruction/disposal.

- **After completion of physical verification of return goods by warehouse and QA,**
  - The Warehouse shall ensure cleaning and/or de-cartooning or redressing (In case of Shipper) of the returned goods as per the condition required.

  - Warehouse personnel shall print "Returned Goods Quarantine label" and shall affix it on each container, based on the recommendation of the Production Head and QA Head.

  - Note: Returned Goods-Quarantine labels shall not be required to affix on the returned container if it is decided to discard the materials.

- QA personnel shall fill the "Returned Goods Verification Report" and forward it to Production Head and QA Head for its recommendation.

- Based on the recommendation of the "Returned Goods Verification Report", return goods are allowed for sampling and reanalysis.

- After reanalysis, if the result complies with the specification limit, then materials shall be released for re-sale after redressing /re-packing.

- If it is failing to meet the specification limit, then material shall be discarded.

- Based on the recommendation of the Production Head and QA Head.

- QA personnel shall forward the "Returned Goods Verification Report".

- QC, in case it is recommended for sampling and reanalysis.

- Packing, in case sampling and reanalysis are not required and material shall directly pack.

- **Warehouse (BSR) in case material is recommended for disposal.**

  - QC Shall generate QC order in the system for sampling and retesting if materials are recommended for reanalysis.

  - QC shall make the entry in Return Goods Verification Report & shall perform sampling and re-testing of returned goods.

  - On completion of reanalysis, QC shall 'Approve' or 'Reject' the material, as appropriate, in system & shall submit all the above documents along-with the analytical documents to QA for further decision.

  - Based on the finding & analytical results of the material, QA shall recommend the action for Redressing/Repacking/Destruction.

  - In the case of sampling and retesting not required of returned goods and it is allowed for Redressing/Repacking directly,

  - Then QA shall forward the Returned Goods Verification Report to the packing department directly.

  - In case if it is decided to reprocess the goods, then it shall be handled through the SOP of "Reprocessing" and the Manufacturing and Expiry date of goods shall remain unchanged.

- **The final disposition of the returned goods shall have to be finalized within 60 days of receipt.**
  - In case if it is decided to disposal the returned goods, then it shall be disposed of as per the SOP "Handling of Rejected Material in Manufacturing Area".

Redressing of Return Goods:

- Packing personnel shall generate the redressing record request after the receipt of Return Goods Verification Report from the QA department.
- Packing personnel shall collect the returned goods from the warehouse (BSR) and store it at an appropriate place before its packing operation.
- QA shall issue the authorized batch redressing record after verifying Manufacturing. Date and Exp. Date.
- Make necessary entries in the same register where previous entry of the same batch is addressed for the issuance.
- The packing officer shall start the commencement of redressing activity after receipt of the batch redressing record.
- Packing personnel shall take the line clearance of area and equipment.
- It shall be recorded in batch redressing records.
- The packing officer and QA officer shall perform the in-process check during the redressing activity.
- Record the same in the batch redressing record.
- After completion of the redressing activity, the QA officer shall withdraw the <u>Control Sample</u> and ensure complete documentation of the batch redressing record.
- After closing of batch redressing record, the QA officer shall fill the final inspection report.
- If found satisfactory shall release the batch for dispatch.
- For any discrepancy found during FP inspection, it shall be discussed with the QA head and corrective action shall be taken as per the recommendation of the QA head.
- QA shall check and review the redressing record and release the batch.

Repacking of Return Goods:

- After the receipt of the Return Goods Verification Report from the QA department.

- Packing personnel shall collect the returned goods from the warehouse (BSR) and store it at the appropriate place before its packing operation.
- Re-packed finished goods shall be assigned batch number which will be suffixed with "R".
- All the packed returned goods shall be defoiled in the environmental controlled area and after defoiling of packed returned goods.
- Packing and QA personnel shall jointly verify the physical condition of defoiled goods for it's repacking.
- On the basis of the physical condition of defoiled goods, QA shall examine the bulk for appearance and decide whether it shall be packed/ discarded.
- If the physical conditions of defoiled goods are not satisfactory, then it shall be allowed for disposal.
- If the physical condition of defoiled goods is satisfactory and it is decided to pack the defoiled goods.
- Then packing personnel shall raise a request to the QA department for issuance of batch packing record.
- QA shall withdraw the sample and send to QC for analysis purpose along with test requisition cum report if required.
- All the defoiled goods containers/carat shall be store in packing quarantine /appropriate place till its commencement of packing activity, with proper status labeling.
- If bulk goods are transferred to the quarantine area then it shall be recorded in the quarantine Inward/Outward Logbook.
- QA officer shall issue the authorized batch packing record after verifying Manufacturing. Date and Exp. Date.
- Make necessary entries in the same register where previous entry of the same batch is addressed for the issuance.

- **The packing officer shall start the commencement of repacking activity after receipt of the batch packing record.**

  - Packing personnel shall take the line clearance of area and equipment as per the Sop.
  - It shall be recorded in the batch packing record.
  - The packing officer and QA officer shall perform the in-process check during the repacking activity,
  - Record the same in the batch packing record.

- After completion of the repacking activity, QA shall ensure complete documentation in the batch packing record and withdraw Control Sample.

- After completion of the packing operation Return Goods Verification Report

- The analytical docket shall be attached with BPR.

- The warehouse shall fill the details in the "Returned goods logbook".

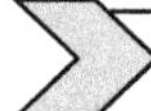 ## 4.3   Recalling

4.3.1   Recall Handling

''Recall'' means a firm's removal or correction of a marketed product that the Food and Drug Administration considers to be in violation of the laws it administers and against which the agency would initiate legal action, e.g., seizure. The main objectives of this recall plan are:

- Stop the distribution and sale of the affected product.

- Effectively notify management, customers and regulatory authority.

- Efficiently remove the affected product from the marketplace, warehouse and/or distribution areas.

- Dispose and conduct a root cause analysis and report the effectiveness and outcome of the recall.

- Implement a corrective action plan to prevent another recall.

4.3.2   SOP on Recall

In case of adverse event a committee evaluates the crisis. It consists of following individuals:

- GM/V.P/QA/QC, Regulatory

- GM Manufacturing

- GM, Formulation and Development

- Medical advisor

- Vice president – Marketing

- Vice president – International Marketing

- Vice president – Technical Operations

4.3.3 Procedure

Any employee becoming aware of such medicine should immediately notify to higher authorities. Immediately quarantine existing in-house of relevant medicine. Record the following information:

(a) The product name, strength, packs size, batch no., manufacturing and expiry date.

(b) The total number of units released for sale.

(c) Date on which distribution commenced.

(d) Total number of units distributed.

(e) Number of units still in stock.

(f) Nature of reported violation.

In the light of above information higher officials evaluates the health hazard presented by the violation medicine and documents it on "medicine recall control document".

The GM, QA/QC Regulatory or GM manufacturing implements recall without delay. They also prepare an interim reconciliation report after 30 days and submit a copy to concerned authorities. After that prepares a final reconciliation report after 90 days and submits a copy for verification of the success of recall.

Signature of GM, QA/QC Regulatory G.M. manufacturing should be taken. Steps should be taken to prevent the re-occurrence. Prior to completion of recall the following points should be considered:

- Method of destruction of the product.

- A designed area to receive returned medicines.

- Inventory of medicine.

- Destruction authorization.

The recall will be terminated when the GM, QA/QC Regulatory or GM manufacturing are assured that recall has been completed reasonably and a "medicine record status report" is completed. GM, QA/QC Regulatory or GM manufacturing shall prepare a "Standardized recall letter" and "press statement". After the authorization by GM, QA/QC Regulatory or GM manufacturing, the recalled material along with stock in hand shall be destroyed and that should be recorded.

4.3.4 Recall Classification

FDA classified the product recall depending on the health hazard caused by the product.

Class I is a situation in which there is a reasonable probability that the use of, or exposure to, a violative product will cause serious adverse health consequences or death.

Class II is a situation in which use of, or exposure to, a violative product may cause temporary or medically reversible adverse health consequences.

Class III is a situation in which use of, or exposure to, a violative product is not likely to cause adverse health consequences.

4.3.5   Recall Policy

Recall is an effective method of removing or correcting consumer products that are in violation of laws administered by the FDA. Recall may be undertaken voluntarily and at any time by manufacturers and distributors, or at the request of FDA. Recall is generally more appropriate and affords better protection for consumers. Seizure, multiple seizure, or other court action is indicated when a firm refuse to undertake a recall requested by the Food and Drug Administration.

4.3.6   Health Hazard Evaluation

An evaluation of the health hazard presented by a product being recalled or considered for recall will be conducted by an ad hoc committee of Food and Drug Administration. It involves the assessment of hazards to various segments of the population, degree of seriousness, likelihood of occurrence, consequences etc.

4.3.7   Recall Team

A recall coordinator is to be appointed and members of a recall team identified from the various functional areas. All members must ensure that all procedures are carried out effectively and efficiently. The team should receive appropriate training. The Recall Management Team list shall be updated at least four times a year.

4.3.8   Recall Strategy

A recall strategy that takes into account the following factors:

   (a)   Results of health hazard evaluation.
   (b)   Ease in identifying the product.
   (c)   Degree to which the products deficiency is obvious to the consumer or user.
   (d)   Degree to which the product remains unused in the market-place.
   (e)   Continued availability of essential products

Elements of a recall strategy:

1. Depth of recall.
2. Public warning.
3. Effectiveness checks:
   - Level A-100 percent of the total number of consignees to be contacted.
   - Level B- greater than 10 percent and less than 100 percent of the total number of consignees.
   - Level C-10 percent of the total number of consignees to be contacted.
   - Level D- 2 percent of the total number of consignees to be contacted.
   - Level E- No effectiveness checks.

4.3.9 Termination of Recall

A recall will be terminated when the FDA is confident that product has been removed from market in accordance with recall strategy. FDA's written notice to the regulate is the real termination.

4.3.10 Product Recall Chart

Assemble the recall management team, Notify health agencies, Identify all products to be recalled, Detain and segregate all products to be recalled which are in the firms control, Prepare the press release, Prepare the continued distribution list.

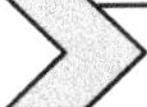 ## 4.4   Waste Disposal

Responsibility: The responsibility may depend on the following of the peoples in the Pharma industry:

- Employees in production unit.
- Representative of QA.
- Housekeeping staff.

4.4.1 Definitions

1. **Scrap**: Materials like rejected foils, bottles, cans, tins etc., which have a resale value and generated at various stages of manufacturing;
   - During compression encapsulation coating & packing stages.
   - In-process check.
   - Rejected printing packing materials.

- From floor sweeping.
- Expired or damaged goods.
- Excess sample in QC after test.
- Product sample from R&D at development stage.

2. **Trash**: This material is to be discarded or disposed by suitable means and don't have a resale value. e.g. dust, unsalable materials

3. **Pharmaceutical Waste:** Pharmaceutical waste is potentially generated thorough a wide variety of activities health care facility general compounding partially used vials syringes, and IV preparation discontinued & unused preparations unused unit dose repacks patients personal medications and outdated pharmaceuticals

4. **Regulatory bodies that oversee pharmaceutical waste management:**
   - Environmental Protection Agency (EPA)
   - Department of Transportation (DOT)
   - Drug Enforcement Administration (DEA)
   - Occupational Safety and Health Administration (OSHA)
   - State Environmental Agencies,
   - State Pharmacy Boards, and
   - Local Publicly Owned Treatment Works (POTW)

4.4.2   Types of Wastes

(a)   On the Bases of State: 1. Solid, 2. Liquid, 3. Gaseous

(b)   On the Base of Effect: 1. Hazardous waste, 2. Bio hazardous waste, 3. Radioactive hazardous waste

(c)   WHO categories of health care waste

1. **Hazardous Waste:** A type of solid wastes that contain substantial or potential threats to public health or the environment. Must meet any of the following criteria:
   - Specifically listed as a hazardous waste by EPA
   - Exhibits one or more of the characteristics of hazardous wastes (ignitability, corrosiveness, reactivity, and/or toxicity)
   - Is generated by the treatment of hazardous waste.

   Storage Requirements: 1) Containers must be in good condition, 2) Containers must be compatible with waste, 3) Containers must be handled in a manner to prevent leaks and spills, 4) Containers must be inspected, 5) Containers must be labeled "Hazardous Waste "and / or list the contents of the container

Characteristic of Hazardous wastes: Characteristic wastes are regulated because they exhibit certain hazardous properties – 1. Ignitability, 2. Corrosivity, 3. Reactivity and 4. Toxicity.

1. **Ignitability**: The objective of the ignitability characteristic is to identify wastes that either present a fire hazard under routine storage, disposal, and transportation or are capable of exacerbating a fire. There are several ways that a drug formulation can exhibit the ignitability characteristic.

2. **Corrosivity**: Any waste which has a pH of less than or equal to 2 (highly acidic) or greater than or equal to12.5 (highly basic) exhibits the characteristic of corrosivity and must be managed as a hazardous waste.

    Generation of corrosive pharmaceutical wastes is generally limited to compounding chemicals in the pharmacy. Compounding chemicals include strong acids, such as glacial acetic acid and strong bases, such as sodium hydroxide.

3. **Reactivity**: Reactive wastes are unstable under "normal" conditions. They can cause explosions, toxic fumes, gases, or vapors when heated, compressed, or mixed with water. Nitroglycerin is the only drug that is potentially reactive.

4. **Toxicity**: Wastes that exceed these concentrations must be managed as hazardous waste. The test that determines the ability of these chemicals and heavy metals to leach in a landfill environment is called the Toxicity Characteristic Leaching Procedure or TCLP. If the concentration determined by the TCLP exceeds the stated limits, the waste must be managed as hazardous waste.

2. **Bio hazardous Waste:** A solid waste that contains or may reasonably be expected to contain pathogens of sufficient virulence and quantity that exposure to the waste by a susceptible host could result in an infectious disease. This waste includes such materials as used sharps (needles, syringes, blades, pipettes, broken glass, and blood vials), body fluids or materials mixed with body fluids, bandages, or other materials that have come in contact with body fluids

Storage Requirements:

*   Containers must be clearly labeled with the international biohazard sign and one of the following: "INFECTIOUS WASTE", "BIOMEDICAL WASTE", or "BIOHAZARD".

*   Sharps must be stored in rigid plastic containers. Other wastes may be stored in plastic bags or rigid containers.

- Labeled with a warning sign consisting of the international biohazard sign "INFECTIOUS WASTE STORAGE AREA" and "UNAUTHORIZED PERSONS KEEP OUT".

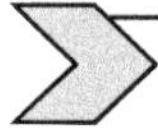 ## 4.5 Document Maintenance in Pharmaceutical Industry

4.5.1 Introduction

Documentation is an integral part of good manufacturing practices. It defines a system of information and control so that risks so inherent in misinterpretation and/or error in oral communication are minimized. It consequently strengthens the quality, and its consistency, of all goods and services, as those responsible for the specific operations have clear, unambiguous instructions to follow including active drug substances, is legally mandatory.

4.5.2 Principle

Documentation is an integral part of good manufacturing practices. It defines a system of information and control so that risks so inherent in misinterpretation and/or error in oral communication are minimized.

It consequently strengthens the quality, and its consistency, of all goods and services, as those responsible for the specific operations have clear, unambiguous instructions to follow including active drug substances, is legally mandatory. (OPPI Guideline)

4.5.3 Objectives of Documents

1. To define the specifications and procedures for all materials and method of manufactured   and control.
2. To ensure that all personal concern with manufacture know what to do and when to do it.
3. To ensure that authorized persons have all the information necessary to decide whether or not to realize a batch of a drug for sale.
4. To ensure the existence of documented evidence, trace ability, and to provide records and an audit trail that will permit investigation.
5. It ensures the availability of the data needed for validation, review and statistical analysis.

4.5.4 Scope

Good documentation encompasses practically all the aspect of pharmaceutical production:

1. **Building and premises:** installation, validation, cleaning and maintenance.
2. **Equipment:** installation, calibration, validation, maintenance, cleaning.
3. **Materials:** specification, testing, ware-housing, use, rejection/disposal.
4. **Processing:** individual steps in the process of manufacturing including controls thereof.
5. **Finished goods:** specifications, testing, storage, distribution, and rejection/disposal.

4.5.5 Characteristic of Document

For effective use of documents, they should be designed and prepared with utmost care. Each document shall:

1. Have a clear title.
2. Have an identification number.
3. Be approved by authorized person.
4. Have the date of issue.
5. Have a due date of revision.
6. List to whom it has been issued.

Where the documents carry instructions (e.g. batch processing)

1. The instructions shall be precise and not ambiguous.
2. They shall be for each individual step and not combined. e.g. Weigh the materials; charge the weighed materials into the blend.
3. Instructions shall be in imperative mood.

Where entry of any data (e.g. temperature, weight) is expected to be made by the person using the document:

1. Sufficient space shall be provided for making the entry.
2. Heading shall clearly indicate what is to be entered, and who is responsible.
3. All entries shall be in ink.
4. All entries shall be clear and legible.
5. Person making the entries shall confirm the entry by initialing/ signing the same.
6. An error in entry shall be so corrected that the original (wrong) entry is not lost. such correction shall also be initialed and dated. Where necessary, reason for correction shall also be recorded, initialed and dated.

Documentation system should provide for a periodic review, and revision, if necessary, of any document, or part thereof. Such revised versions shall also be approved by the authorized persons.

Outdate/superseded document shall be immediately removed from active use, and copy retained only for reference. If documentation is through electronic data processing system (computerized system) there shall be adequate, reliable systems in place:

1. To check and ensure correctness of data.

2. To record changes (addition/deletion)

3. That meets other regulation requirement, if any.

For implementing efficient documentation practices, which meet, full GLP/GMP/ISO and FDA requirements. Here is a hint from the "documents" model, which lists out the areas required for GMP document implementation:

D = Design, development, deviations, dossiers and Drug Master Files for regulated markets, distribution records

O = Operational procedures/techniques/methods, Out of specifications (OOS), Out of trend (OOT)

C = Cleaning, calibration, controls, complaints, containers and closures, contamination and change control

U = User requirement specifications, utilities like water systems, HVAC, AHU etc.

M = Man, materials, machines, methods, maintenance, manufacturing operations and controls, monitoring, master formula, manuals (quality, safety and environment), medical records

E = Engineering control and practices, Environment control, Equipment qualification documents

N = Non-routine activities, New products and substances

T = Technology transfer, training, testing, Trend analysis, Technical dossiers

S = SOPs, safety practices, sanitation, storage, self-inspection, standardization, supplier qualification, specifications and standard test procedures and site master file. (Quality Assurance)

4.5.6 Types of Documentation

Documentation may be divided into:

1. **Documents:** Procedural or instructional documentation.

   Benefits:

   - Reference for future use or a means to communicate information to others.

- Particularly important to ensure that knowledge is not lost when employee leaves.
- Ensure the quality and consistency of processed/ activities/ manufacturing.

2. **Records:** Evidence of compliance

   Benefits:
   - Provide background history.
   - Protects intellectual property (Evidence of an idea or a finding including the date and the responsible person).
   - Provide legally valid evidence.

4.5.7 Batch Formula Record

Batch manufacturing record is a written document of the batch, prepared during pharmaceutical manufacturing process. Batch manufacturing record is like a proof that batches were properly made and checked by quality control personnel. It contains actual data and step by step process for manufacturing each batch.

Batch manufacturing record is like a proof that batches were properly made and checked by quality control personnel. This ensures that proper ingredients are added and each processing step is completed according to the SOP and also ensures uniformity in finished product in each batch.

BMR (Batch Manufacturing Record) is one of the key documents in pharmaceutical. It is a record or history for every batch manufactured in pharmaceuticals.

BMR is called as by followings too:
- BPR-Batch processing record
- BPCR -Batch processing & control record
- BMR with BPR-Batch manufacturing & Batch packaging record etc

Batch manufacturing & batch packaging record is itself a documentary for a particular product manufacturing in pharmaceutical plant which have a sequential data recording along with facility, utility and product parameters.

4.5.7.1 Preparation of Batch Manufacturing & Batch Packaging Record

- Batch manufacturing & batch packaging record shall be prepared for each product or by following suitability, in easy language we can say each product have their own BMR.
- BMR & BPR is prepared by user, and user is production personnel, prepared by production personnel and then shall be checked by production head and after that reviewed by QA. BMR & BPR shall be

prepared by following step of master formula record given by R&D (research & development) or PDD (Product development department).

- After reviewed by QA final print of BMR shall be taken out by QA, and all related signature shall be done.

- Signed copy stamped by master copy stamp in a designated place in BMR and then kept in lock and key by QA.

- Master copy shall be photocopied after getting BMR & BPR requisition by production department. Photocopied BMR shall stamped by controlled copy and same shall be send to production.

- Issuance of BMR & BPR shall maintain in a issuance register and receiving shall be taken by production personnel as a proof of issuance.

4.5.7.2 Usage of Batch Manufacturing & Batch Packaging Record

- Production personnel shall start to write on the same from when they shall start dispensing of that particular product.

- All stages recording from starting to end, dispensing to dispatch should cover in BMR & BPR.

- All related personnel shall sign off after doing data recording including IPQA, each stage verification and line clearance shall denote the product progress.

- When a step completed practically in shop floor that should be also finished in BMR. Online filling of BMR & BPR is must.

- One stage completing product and BMR shall transfer to next stage, before line clearance production personnel and IPQA shall ensure the completeness of previous step.

- In case of discrepancy in last step of production, production shall be stopped and should start after rectification of same.

- At stage of packing product's final analysis-Finished goods analysis shall completed by QC, and then complete BMR shall reviewed by QA before final release of product.

- After final review if everything is clear and correct than QA shall release the finished product and BMR shall close for the same.

- Closed BMR & BPR shall deposit in document cell in QA.

- A log for deposition of all BMR & BPR shall maintained by Documentation cell incharge in QA.

- In case, review of previous batch to be done, issuance of previous BMR shall too log in Deposition register.

- After completion of retention period i.e. 5 years or product expiry plus one whatever is greater (as per WHO), destruction of BMR & BPR shall be done by following destruction policy of organization and record shall maintained accordingly.

* Destruction shall be done by QA.

4.5.8 Master Formula Record

Master formula record is a product specific document compiled, checked, authorized and approved by competent technical personnel from different. But interlinked, functions such as development, production, packaging and quality control as necessary and appropriate.

As with any other documentation master formula record shall also be open for review. Changes, if any shall also be approved by designated persons responsible for production and quality control.

Master formula record shall:

(a) Give patent/proprietary name of the product, and its strength.

(b) Give pharmacopoeial/generic name of the product, and its strength.

(c) Give dosage form (e.g. tablet, ampoule) and physical characteristics of the product.

(d) Give sufficient, detailed information of product pack and primary packaging materials.

(e) Give identity, quality and quantity of every ingredient, including overages/assay value-based quantities, if any, irrespective of whether, or not, the material.

(f) Briefly describe all raw materials.

(g) Give broad outlines of the process of manufacture (as a flow-chart, for example).

(h) Give brief description of equipment/ machinery used for manufacturing the product.

(i) Give step-wise manufacturing process.

(j) Give theoretical and practical (expected) yields at different stages of manufacture.

(k) Bring out in sufficient details precautions to be taken during manufacturing to ensure birth product quality and personnel safety.

(l) Give all analytical controls, including limits thereof, applicable to the finished product.

(m) Give stability test results covering the assigned shelf life.

(n) Have a 'product history' data giving references in manufacturing/ packaging introduced over the year.

(o) (Preferably) contain samples of printed packaging components.

4.5.9   SOP

A Standard Operating Procedure (SOP) is a set of written instructions that document a routine or repetitive activity which is followed by employees in an organization. The development and use of SOPs are an integral part of a successful quality system. It provides information to perform a job properly, and consistently in order to achieve pre-determined specification and quality endresult. SOPs should allow for the continual improvement of standards of service, and provide evidence of commitment towards protecting patients. Additional benefits are: Help to assure quality and consistency of service; Help to ensure that good practice is achieved at all times; Provide an opportunity to fully utilize the expertise of all team members; Enable pharmacists to delegate; Help to avoid confusion over who does what (role clarification); Provide advice and guidance to locums and part-time staff; They are useful tools for training new members of staff; Provide a contribution to the audit process.

4.5.9.1   Benefits of SOP

To provide people with all the safety, health, environmental and operational information necessary to perform a job properly. Placing value only on production while ignoring safety, health and environment is costly in the long run. It is better to train employees in all aspects of doing a job than to face accidents, fines and litigation later.

To ensure that production operations are performed consistently to maintain quality control of processes and products. Consumers, from individuals to companies, want products of consistent quality and specifications. SOPs specify job steps that help standardize products and therefore quality. To ensure that processes continue uninterrupted and are completed on a prescribed schedule. By following SOPs, you help ensure against process shut-downs caused by equipment failure or other facility damage. To ensure that no failures occur in manufacturing and other processes that would harm anyone in the surrounding community. Following health and environmental steps in SOPs ensures against spills and emissions that threaten plant neighbors and create community outrage.

Properly maintained written SOPs can chronicle the best knowledge that can serve new workers when older ones move on. To serve as an explanation of steps in a process so they can be reviewed in accident investigations.

- Although accidents are unfortunate, view them as opportunities to learn how to improve conditions. A good SOP gives you a basis from which to being investigating accidents. Ten reasons for writing SOPs: To provide individuals who perform operations with all the safety, health, environmental and operational information required to perform a job properly. To protect the health and safety of employees, and to protect the environment.

- To protect the community.

4.5.9.2 SOP Process

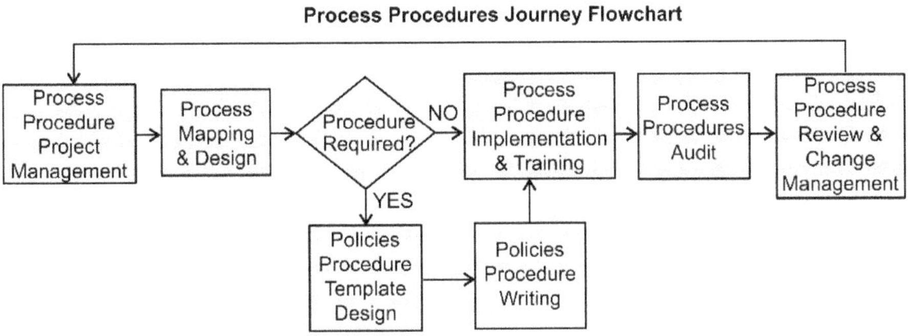

Process Procedures Journey Flowchart

Process Procedure Project Management → Process Mapping & Design → Procedure Required? — NO → Process Procedure Implementation & Training → Process Procedures Audit → Process Procedure Review & Change Management

Procedure Required? — YES → Policies Procedure Template Design → Policies Procedure Writing → Process Procedure Implementation & Training

Figure 4.1 SOP Process.

4.5.9.3 SOP Preparation

The organization should have a procedure in place for determining what procedures or processes need to be documented. Those SOPs should then be written by individuals knowledgeable with the activity and the organization's internal structure. These individuals are essentially subject matter experts who actually perform the work or use the process. A team approach can be followed, especially for multi-tasked processes where the experiences of a number of individuals are critical, which also promotes "buy-in" from potential users of the SOP. SOPs should be written with sufficient detail so that someone with limited experience with or knowledge of the procedure, but with a basic understanding, can successfully reproduce the procedure when unsupervised.

The experience requirement for performing an activity should be noted in the section on personnel qualifications. For example, if a basic chemistry or biological course experience or additional training is required that requirement should be indicated. SOP Review and Approval SOPs should be reviewed (that is, validated) by one or more individuals with appropriate training and experience with the process. It is especially helpful if draft SOPs are actually tested by individuals other than the original writer before the SOPs are finalized. The finalized SOPs should be approved as described in the organization's Quality Management Plan or its own SOP for preparation of SOPs. Generally, the immediate supervisor, such as a section or branch chief, and the organization's quality assurance officer review and approve each SOP. Signature approval indicates that an SOP has been both reviewed and approved by management. As per the Government Paperwork Elimination Act of 1998, use of electronic signatures, as well as electronic maintenance and submission, is an acceptable substitution for paper, when practical.

Frequency of Revisions and Reviews: SOPs need to remain current to be useful. Therefore, whenever procedures are changed, SOPs should be updated and re-approved. If desired, modify only the pertinent section of an SOP and indicate the change date/revision number for that section in the Table of contents and the document control notation. SOPs should be also systematically reviewed on a periodic basis, e.g. every 1-2 years, to ensure that the policies and procedures remain current and appropriate, or to determine whether the SOPs are even needed. The review date should be added to each SOP that has been reviewed. If an SOP describes a process that is no longer followed, it should be withdrawn from the current file and archived. Checklists Many activities use checklists to ensure that steps are followed in order.

Checklists are also used to document completed actions. Any checklists or forms included as part of an activity should be referenced at the points in the procedure where they are to be used and then attached to the SOP. In some cases, detailed checklists are prepared specifically for a given activity. In those cases, the SOP should describe, at least generally, how the checklist is to be prepared, or on what it is to be based. Copies of specific checklists should be then maintained in the file with the activity results and/or with the SOP. Remember that the checklist is not the SOP, but a part of the SOP.

Document Control: Each organization should develop a numbering system to systematically identify and label their SOPs, and the document control should be described in its Quality Management Plan. Generally, each page of an SOP should have control documentation notation, similar to that illustrated below. A short title and identification (ID) number can serve as a reference designation. The revision number and date are very useful in identifying the SOP in use when reviewing historical data and is critical when the need for evidentiary records is involved and when the activity is being reviewed. When the number of pages is indicated, the user can quickly check if the SOP is complete. Generally, this type of document control notation is located in the upper right-hand corner of each document page following the title page.

SOP Document Tracking and Archival: The organization should maintain a master list of all SOPs. This file or database should indicate the SOP number, version number, date of issuance, title, author, status, organizational division, branch, section, and any historical information regarding past versions. The QA Manager (or designee) is generally the individual responsible for maintaining a file listing all current quality-related SOPs used within the organization. If an electronic database is used, automatic "Review SOP" notices can be sent. Note that this list may be used also when audits are being considered or when questions are raised as to practices being followed within the organization.

4.5.10 Quality Audit

Auditing in simple terms could be defined as inspection of a process or a system to make sure that it complies with the requirements of its intended use.

In pharmaceutical industry audits are virtual means to evaluate compliance with the set objectives as defined in the quality system and thereby paving a path of continuous improvement program by giving the feedback to the management.

There are two types of audits that are conducted:
1. **Internal Audit (Self Inspection):** This is conducted within the premises to monitor the implementation and respect of good manufacturing practices. This is also done to have prior information about the flaws in the system and taking necessary corrective and preventive measures.
2. **External Audit:** This is conducted for the suppliers or any outsourcing operations carried out by the pharmaceutical industry. The contract giver (Industry) is responsible to access the competence of the Contract acceptor (supplier or any other outsource operations department) as per the GMP guidelines.

4.5.10.1 Procedure for Conducting an Audit

It is mandatory that there should be a well written procedure for conducting an audit whether it is an internal or external audit. The procedure should begin with a clear objective that why an audit is being conducted. Other important point that must be described are as follows:
1. **Frequency of Audit:** The procedure how frequency of audit must be defined and as per that frequency must be set and followed accordingly.
2. **Responsibilities:** The audit team must be defined that will be responsible for conducting and reviewing the audit reports. The people in the audit team must be well equipped with the operations and procedures that are being audited.
3. **Documentation:** It is important to document each and every audit conducted as it not only helps from regulatory perspective but also act as reference document to have a insight of flaws previously faced.

4.5.10.2 Audit Preparation

The audit must be initiated with an agenda that gives a real time frame to all the parties involved. This is done so that all the personnel involved, documentation and everything else is available at the required time.

The proposed agenda must be agreed through a pre-planned meeting and sorted out all the other requirements that must be required at the time of the audit (from a simple schedule detail to complex documentation).

Next audit checklist must be created that prevent unnecessary time wastage in reading big paragraphs. The checklist must be framed according to the type of the audit being conducted and procedures and policies to be audited.

4.5.10.3 Conducting of Audit

1. The audit team must abide rules and regulations that are specific to the operations that are carried out at the premises. For example: if the audit is conducted in aseptic section it is mandatory to put the safety clothing as per cGMP that is must for everyone who so ever enter that portion.

2. The audit must be done by communicating by the audit team with the personnel working and all the findings must be documented. But it is also important to explain the observations that make it more realistic rather than just noting it down and explaining later on.

3. The audit team must be flexible. The procedure to meet the requirements of GMP could be different in different industries hence the auditor must focus on the results and then decide about the observations.

4. The conclusions obtained must be prepared, documented and finally completed as a audit report.

4.5.10.4 Completing and Follow up of Audit

There should be a close out meeting after the conduct of the audit. The observations that are made and recorded should be clear to both the parties (auditor and auditee) as the commitments has to be made for corrective actions to be taken. For this the schedules are made to take the corrective actions against the observations made and through that follow up of audit is done. There might be some unusual activities found during the audit, for those preventive measures must be conducted to avoid any findings again.

4.5.11 Quality Documentation

Appropriate, Adequate, Accurate and Current

The word "documentation" encompasses both records and documents. Records are recorded information, regardless of the medium or characteristics, made or received by an organization that is useful in the operation of the organization. They are also any information captured in reproducible form that is required for conducting business. Documents, on the other hand, is a term that denotes written or graphical procedures, policies or instructions. Documents explain what an organization plans to do and how it will be accomplished as well as instruct employees how to perform tasks. Unlike records, documents exist before the fact; they provide guidelines, explanations and instructions about how to operate. Records contain information about the activity and, thus, do not exist until after the activity has been performed. Documents include quality manuals, raw materials specifications and procedures on such topics as internal quality audits, marketing, quality control, hazardous waste handling, document control, etc.

The benefits to the audit of properly maintaining organizational records and documents should be obvious. First, properly maintained documentation provides employees with the official "company way" of performing their tasks as related to ensuring product quality. Next, documentation can be very useful in simplifying complex (and, thereby, error-prone) processes. Documentation can be used to supplement employee training. It provides a basis for comparing what is required to what is actually done. Documentation, in other words, can be audited to verify compliance. It is an excellent source of objective evidence for the auditor. Documentation also provides a method of evaluating the quality system per-formance of suppliers and sub-tier suppliers to ensure the best provider of quality material and products is selected.

The GDP can be defined as "Good documentation practice is an essential part of the quality assurance and such, related to all aspects of GMP" this definition is based on WHO. Clearly written documents prevent errors of various activities in pharma each and every activity is written in specific documents such as SOPs and strictly followed.

Spoken communications may be create errors so that all important documents such as Master formula record, procedure and record must be free from errors and documented.

It is difficult to make a list of required documents and totally depend upon Companies activity or environment. Followings are the activity factors considered during designing of any documents.

1. Type of formulation
2. Country requirements
3. Availability of ERP or SAP system

4.5.11.1 Purpose of Documentations

- Defines specifications and procedures for all materials and methods of manufacture and control

- Ensures all personnel know what to do and when to do it
- Ensure that authorized persons have all information necessary for release of product
- Ensures documented evidence, traceability, provide records and audit trail for investigation
- Ensures availability of data for validation, review and statistical analysis.

4.5.11.2 Quality Review

Product Quality Review is regular periodic or rolling quality reviews of all licensed medicinal products, including export only products, which are conducted with the objective of verifying the consistency of the existing process, the appropriateness of current specifications for both starting materials and finished product to highlight any trends and to identify product and process improvements. The Product Quality review (PQR) is an effective quality improvement tool to enhance the consistency of the process and the overall quality of the product. The PQR will capture a broader view of product data, capturing trends and will help determine the need for revalidation and changes, if any.

4.5.11.3 Procedure

Product Quality Review should typically be carried out for each product manufactured in the previous year. In the case of campaign manufacturing, the review period can be extended beyond a year. Such extensions shall be for a limited number of months and as described in a procedure.

Along with PQR, implementation of preceding years' recommendations shall be reviewed. The Product Quality Review Report should contain at least the following details:

(i) A review of starting materials and product contact primary packaging materials used for the product, especially those from new sources.

   (a) Summary of all batches of starting and packaging materials received in a year and their approval status;

   (b) Summary of the suppliers/manufacturers of the materials;

   (c) Compilation and analysis of the results of analytical tests for key quality attributes such as description, identification, loss on drying/water content by Karl Fisher, particle size, related substances and assay;

   (d) Compilation of the Certificate of analysis (COA) results obtained from supplier/manufacturer, if the batch is released based on supplier's COA.

(e) Summary of details related to any significant deviations observed such as rejection of vendor lots.

(ii) A review of critical in-process controls and finished product results. (a) Compilation(s) and analysis of in-process test results obtained from the total number of batches manufactured in that particular year e.g. weight variation, dimension, friability, hardness, disintegration time, fill volume variation (such as for ampoules, vials, bottles), pH, etc (b) Compilation(s) and analysis of finished product test results such as description/appearance, identification, pH, loss on drying/Water by KF, viscosity, dissolution test, impurities and related substances, degradation product (if any) and assay.

(iii) A review of all batches that failed to meet established specification(s) and their investigation.

4.5.12 Distribution Records

- Distribution records shall contain the name and strength of the product and description of the dosage form, name and address of the consignee, date and quality shipped, and lot or control number of the drug product. For compressed medical gas products, distribution records are not required to contain lot or control numbers.

- The primary purpose is to ensure that adequate data are available to access trade customers should a recall be initiated. The recording of lot number to each order will certainly accomplish this purpose.

- The recordings of dates on which a specific lot of product commenced and ceased distribution may be used. All customers receiving the product between these dates could then be contacted.

- Obviously on the first and last days of distribution, some of the customers may have received product from the end of previous lot or the beginning of the next lot.

- This overlap should in no way adversely impact on the effectiveness of a recall.

- Whatever system is used, it must accommodate the reintroduction of returned goods into the distribution chain.

- Distribution records include a wide range of documentation such as invoices, bills of lading, customers' receipts, internal warehouse storage and inventory records.

- The information required need not be on every document. Also, customer codes and product codes may be used as alternates to customer names and address and product names.

4.5.12.1 Reports and Documents

- The management of each operational site is required to define responsibility for origination, distribution, maintenance, change control, and archiving of all GMP documentation and records within that department or unit.

- Document owners are required to ensure that all aspects of documentation and records management specified in form of standard operating procedures (SOPs).

- All associates have the responsibility of ensuring that all GMP activities are performed according to the official SOPs; any deviations in procedure are reported to their supervisor and are adequately documented.

- The local quality assurance unit has the responsibility of ensuring via organizational measures and auditing that GMP documentation and records systems used within the operational unit are complete and comply with the relevant GMP requirements, and also that the requirements of the SOPs are followed.

- Requirements for specific documents or record, including ownership, content, authorization, and change control procedures, has to be described or cross-referenced in the quality modules which relate to the subject of the document.

- Good documentation constitutes an essential part of the quality assurance system. Clearly written procedures prevent errors resulting from spoken communication, and clear documentation permits tracing of activities performed.

- Documents must be designed, prepared, reviewed, and distributed with care.

- Documents must be approved, signed, and dated by the appropriate competent and authorized persons.

- Documents must have unambiguous contents. The title, nature, and purpose should be clearly stated. They must be laid out in an orderly fashion and be easy to check. Reproduced documents must be clear and legible.

- Documents must be regularly reviewed and kept up-to-date. When a document has been revised, systems must be operated to prevent inadvertent use of superseded documents (e.g., only current documentation should be available for use).

- Documents must not be handwritten; however, where documents require the entry of data, these entries may be made in clear legible handwriting using a suitable indelible medium (i.e., not a pencil). Sufficient space must be provided for such entries.

- Any correction made to a document or record must be signed or initialed and dated; the correction must permit the reading of the original information. Where appropriate, the reason for the correction must be recorded.

- Record must be kept at the time each action is taken and in such a way that all activities concerning the conduct of preclinical studies, clinical trials, and the manufacture and control of products are traceable. • Storage of critical records must at secure place, with access limited to authorized persons. The storage location must ensure adequate protection from loss, destruction, or falsification, and from damage due to fire, water, etc.

- Records which are critical to regulatory compliance or to support essential business activities must be duplicated on paper, microfilm, or electronically, and stored in a separate, secure location in a separate building from the originals.

- Date may be recorded by electromagnetic or photographic means, but detailed procedures relating to whatever system is adopted must be available. Accuracy of the record should be checked as per the defined procedure. If documentation is handled by electronic data processing methods, only authorized persons should be able to enter or modify data in the computer, access must be restricted by passwords or other means, and entry of critical data must be independently checked.

- It is particularly important that during the period of retention, the data can be rendered legible within an appropriate period of time.

- If data is modified, it must be traceable.

There are various types of procedures that a GMP facility can follow. Given below is a list of the most common types of documents, along with a brief description of each.

1. **Quality manual:** A global company document that describes, in paragraph form, the regulations and/or parts of the regulations that the company is required to follow.

2. **Policies:** Documents that describe in general terms, and not with step-by-step instructions, how specific GMP aspects (such as security, documentation, health, and responsibilities) will be implemented.

3. **Standard operating procedures (SOPs):** Step-by-step instructions for performing operational tasks or activities.

4. **Batch records:** These documents are typically used and completed by the manufacturing department. Batch records provide step-by-step

instructions for production-related tasks and activities, besides including areas on the batch record itself for documenting such tasks.

5. **Test methods:** These documents are typically used and completed by the quality control (QC) department. Test methods provide step-by-step instructions for testing supplies, materials, products, and other production-related tasks and activities, e.g., environmental monitoring of the GMP facility.

Specifications: Documents that list the requirements that a supply, material, or product must meet before being released for use or sale. The QC department will compare their test results to specifications to determine if they pass the test.

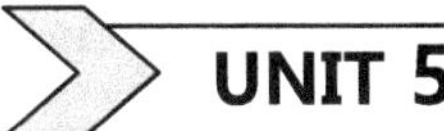

UNIT 5

Calibration and Validation

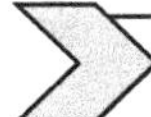

5.1 Validation

Validation is an integral part of quality assurance; it involves the systematic study of systems, facilities and processes aimed at determining whether they perform their intended functions adequately and consistently as specified.

A validated process is one which has been demonstrated to provide a high degree of assurance that uniform batches will be produced that meet the required specifications and has therefore been formally approved.

Validation in itself does not improve processes but confirms that the processes have been properly developed and are under control.

5.1.1 Definitions

- According to **ISO:**

  "Validation is the **confirmation by examination** and the provision of objective evidence that the particular requirements for a specific intended use are fulfilled."

- According to the **US Food and Drug Administration (FDA),** the goal of validation is to:

  "Establish documented evidence which **provides a high degree of assurance** that a specific process will consistently produce a product **meeting its predetermined specifications and quality attributes.**"

- According to **European commission:**

  "Action providing in accordance with the principles of GMP, that any procedure, process, equipment, material, activity or system actually lead to the expected results."

5.1.2 Principle

- Qualification and Validation: Essential part of GMP.

- Manufacturer has to identify what qualification and validation work is required.
- Provides proof that critical aspects of work are controlled and provide documented evidence.
- Key elements of qualification and validation defined and documented: Policy and approach.

5.1.3 Scope of Validation

- Validation requires an appropriate and sufficient infrastructure including organization, documentation, personnel and finances.
- Involvement of management and quality assurance personnel.
- Personnel with appropriate qualifications and experience.
- Extensive preparation and planning before validation is performed.
- Validation should be performed:
    (a) for new premises, equipment, utilities and systems, and processes and procedures;
    (b) at periodic intervals; and
    (c) when major changes have been made.
- Validation in accordance with written protocols.
- Validation over a period of time, e.g. at least three consecutive batches (full production scale) to demonstrate consistency. (Worst case situations should be considered.)
- Significant changes (facilities, equipment, processes) - should be validated
- Risk assessment approach used to determine the scope and extent of validation needed.

5.1.4   Importance of Validation

1. Assurance of quality
2. Time bound
3. Process optimization
4. Reduction of quality cost
5. Nominal mix-ups
6. Minimal batch failures, improved efficiently and productivity
7. Reduction in rejections
8. Increased output
9. Avoidance of capital expenditures
10. Fewer complaints about process related failures

11. Reduced testing in process and in finished good

12. More rapid and reliable start-up of new equipment

13. Easier scale-up form development work

14. Easier maintenance of equipment

15. Improved employee awareness of processes

16. More rapid automation

17. Government regulation (Compliance with validation requirements is necessary for obtaining approval to manufacture and to introduce new products)

5.1.5 Phases in Process Validation

The activities relating to validation studies may be classified into three phases:

Phase 1- Pre-validation phase or the qualification phase, which covers all activities relating to product research and development, formulation, pilot batch studies, scale-up studies, transfer of technology to commercial scale batches, establishing stability conditions, storage and handling of in-process and finished dosage forms, equipment qualification, installation qualification, master production documents, operational qualification, process capability.

Phase 2- Process validation phase (Process Qualification phase) designed to verify that all established limits of the critical process parameters are valid and that satisfactory products can be produced even under the "worst case" conditions.

Phase 3- Validation maintenance phase requiring frequent review of all process related documents, including validation audit reports to assure that there have been no changes, deviations, failures, modifications to the production process, and that all SOPs have been followed, including change control procedures.

5.1.6 Planning for Validation

- The key elements of a validation program should be clearly defined and documented in a validation master plan (VMP) or equivalent documents.

- The VMP should be a summary document, which is brief, concise and clear.

The VMP should contain data on at least the following:

1. Validation policy.

2. Organizational structure of validation activities.

3. Summary of facilities, systems, equipment and processes to be validated.

4. Documentation format: The format to be used for protocols and reports.

5. Planning and scheduling.

6. Change control.

7. Reference to existing document.

8. In case of large projects, it may be necessary to create separate validation master plans.

5.1.7 Documentation

- A written protocol should be established that specifies how qualification and validation will be conducted.

- The protocol should be reviewed and approved.

- The protocol should specify critical steps and acceptance criteria.

- A report that cross-references the qualification and/or validation protocol should be prepared, summarizing the results obtained, commenting on any deviations observed, and drawing the necessary conclusions, including recommending changes necessary to correct deficiencies.

- A written protocol should be established that specifies how qualification and validation will be conducted.

- The protocol should be reviewed and approved.

- The protocol should specify critical steps and acceptance criteria.

- A report that cross-references the qualification and/or validation protocol should be prepared, summarizing the results obtained, commenting on any deviations observed, and drawing the necessary conclusions, including recommending changes necessary to correct deficiencies.

5.1.8 Types of Validation

- Prospective validation
- Concurrent Validation
- Retrospective Validation

5.1.8.1 Prospective Validation

- It is defined as the established documented evidence that a system does what it significances to do based on a pre-planned protocol.

- This validation usually carried out prior to distribution either of a new product or a product made under a revised manufacturing process.

Performed on at least three successive production-size (Consecutive batches).

- In Prospective Validation, the validation protocol is executed before the process is put into commercial use.

- During the product development phase, the production process should be categorized into individual steps.

- Each step should be evaluated on the basis of experience or theoretical considerations to determine the critical parameters that may affect the quality of the finished product.

- A series of experiment should be designed to determine the criticality of these factors.

- All equipment, production environment and the analytical testing methods to be used should have been fully validated.

- Master batch documents can be prepared only after the critical parameters of the process have been identified and machine settings, component specifications and environmental conditions have been determined.

- Using this defined process a series of batches should be produced. In theory, the number of process runs carried out and observations made should be sufficient to allow the normal extent of variation and trends to be established to provide sufficient data for evaluation.

- It is generally considered acceptable that three consecutive batches/runs within the finally agreed parameters, giving product of the desired quality would constitute a proper validation of the process.

Some considerations should be exercised when selecting the process validation strategy.

- The use of different lots of active raw materials and major excipients.

- Batches produced on different shifts.

- The use of different equipment and facilities dedicated for commercial production.

- Operating range of the critical processes.

- A thorough analysis of the process data in case of requalification and revalidation.

- During the processing of the validation batches, extensive sampling and testing should be performed on the product at various stages, and should be documented comprehensively.

- Detailed testing should also be done on the final product in its package.

- Upon completion of the review, recommendations should be made on the extent of monitoring and the in-process controls necessary for routine production.

- These should be incorporated into the Batch manufacturing and packaging record or into appropriate standard operating procedures.

- Limits, frequencies and action to be taken in the event of the limits being exceeded should be specified.

5.1.8.2 Concurrent Validation

- It is similar to prospective, except the operating firm will sell the product during the qualification runs, to the public at its market price, and also similar to retrospective validation.

- This validation involves in-process monitoring of critical processing steps and product testing.

- This helps to generate and documented evidence to show that the production process is in a state of control.

- In exceptional circumstances it may be acceptable not to complete a validation program before routine production starts.

- The decision to carry out concurrent validation must be justified, documented and approved by authorized personnel.

- Documentation requirements for concurrent validation are the same as specified for prospective validation.

5.1.8.3 Retrospective Validation

- It is defined as the established documented evidence that a system does what it purports to do on the review and analysis of historical information.

- This is achieved by the review of the historical manufacturing testing data to prove that the process has always remained in control.

- This type of validation of a process for a product already in distribution.

- Retrospective validation is only acceptable for well-established processes and will be inappropriate where there have been recent changes in the composition of the product, operating procedures or equipment.

- The steps involved require the preparation of a specific protocol and the reporting of the results of the data review, leading to a conclusion and a recommendation.

- For retrospective validation, generally data from ten to thirty consecutive batches should be examined to access process consistency, but fewer batches may be examined if justified.

The source of data for **Retrospective** validation:

- Batch processing and packaging records
- Process control charts
- Maintenance logbooks
- Records of personnel changes
- Process capability studies
- Finished product data
- Storage stability results
- Batches selected for retrospective validation should be representative of all batches made during the review period, including any batches that failed to meet the specifications, and should be sufficient in number to demonstrate process consistency.

5.1.9   Change Control

Written procedures should be in place to describe the actions to be taken if change is proposed to

- Starting material
- Product component
- Process equipment
- Process environment (or site)
- Method of production or testing or any other change that may affect product quality or reproducibility of the process.
- Change control procedure should ensure that sufficient support data are generated to demonstrate that the revised process will result in a product of the desired quality, consistent with the approved specifications.
- All changes that may affect product quality or reproducibility of the process should be formally requested, documented and accepted.
- The likely impact of the change of facilities, systems and equipment on the product should be evaluated, including risk analysis.
- The need for, and the extent of, requalification and revalidation should be determined.

5.1.10 Revalidation

- Re-validation provides the evidence that changes in a process and/or the process environment that are introduced do not adversely affect process characteristics and product quality.
- Documentation requirements will be the same as for the initial validation of the process.

- Facilities, systems, equipment and processes, including cleaning, should be periodically evaluated to confirm that they remain valid.

- Where no significant changes have been made to the validated status, a review with evidence that facilities, systems, equipment and processes meet the prescribed requirements fulfils the need for revalidation.

Some of the changes that require validation are as follows:

- Changes in raw materials (physical properties such as density, viscosity, particle size distribution and moisture etc., that may affect the process or product).

- Changes in the source of active raw material manufacturer.

- Changes in packaging material (primary container/closure system).

- Changes in the process (e.g., mixing time, drying temperatures and batch size).

- Changes in the equipment (e.g., addition of automatic detection system).

- Changes of equipment which involve the replacement of equipment on a "like for like" basis would not normally require re-validation except that this new equipment must be qualified.

- Changes in the plant/facility.

- A decision not to perform revalidation studies must be fully justified and documented.

5.1.11 Validation Master Plan (VMP)

A "Validation Master Plan (VMP)" is a document that summarizes the manufacturer's overall philosophy, intentions and approach to be used for establishing performance adequacy. The following slides review the nature and extent of the contents of the VMP and what the manufacturer's strategy should be.

- Philosophy
- Content
- Strategy

The VMP helps:

- Management
- Validation team members
- Project leaders
- GMP inspectors
- Identifies validation items (products, processes, systems)

- Defines nature and extent of testing expected
- Outlines test procedures and protocols
- Summary document
- Management agreement

Validation activities in VMP

- Every validation activity included
- Revalidation
- Validation of new process cycles
- Large validation projects have separate VMPs
- Include reasonable unexpected events

The VMP

- Enables overview of entire validation project
- Lists items to be validated with the planning schedule as its heart is like a map

The "Introduction" to the VMP

- Validation policy
- Project scope
- Location and timing (including priorities)
- Validation procedures
- Standards

VMP should state who is responsible for:

- Preparing the VMP
- The protocols and SOPs
- Validation work
- Report and document preparation and control
- Approval/authorisation of validation protocols and reports in all stages of validation process
- Tracking system
- Training needs in support of validation

VMP should contain

- Cross references to documents
- Specific process considerations
- Specific characteristics briefly outlined
- Validation list (What to validate)

> Premises, systems and equipment
> Processes
> Products

- Descriptions of plant (where to validate) processes and products
- Personnel attributes such as expertise and training
- Key acceptance criteria
- Format for protocols and other documentation
- List of relevant SOPs (How)
- Planning and scheduling (When)
- Location (Where)
- Estimate of staffing requirements (Who)
- A time plan of the project (When)
- Annexes

In summary, a VMP should contain at least:
- Validation policy
- Organizational structure
- Summary of facilities, systems, equipment, processes to be validated
- Documentation format for protocols and reports
- Planning and scheduling
- Change control
- Training requirements

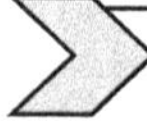

5.2   Analytical Method Validation

Analytical Procedure
- The analytical procedure refers to the way of performing the analysis.
- It should describe in detail the steps necessary to perform each analytical test.
- Component

The sample, the reference standard and the reagents preparations, use of the apparatus, generation of the calibration curve, use of the formulae for the calculation, etc.

Definition

Analytical method validation is the process of demonstrating that analytical procedures are suitable for their intended use and that they support the identity, strength, quality, purity and potency of the drug substances and drug products.

The objective of validation of an analytical procedure is to demonstrate that it is suitable for its intended purpose.

Types of Analytical Procedures to be Validated

- Identification tests
- Quantitative tests for impurities content
- Limit tests for the control of impurities
- Quantitative tests of the active moiety in samples of drug substance or drug product or other selected component(s) in the drug product
- Bioanalytical procedure

5.2.1   Different Principle of Analytical Method Validation

1. Specificity / Selectivity

- Specificity is the ability to assess unequivocally the analyte in the presence of components which may be expected to be present. Typically these might include impurities, degradants, matrix, etc.
- Analyses of blank samples from different subjects (n=6) for interference using the proposed extraction procedure and other chromatographic conditions.
- Results should be compared with those obtained with aqueous solution of the analyte at a concentration near the LOQ.
- An investigation of specificity should be conducted during the validation of identification tests, the determination of impurities and the assay.
- It is not always possible to demonstrate that an analytical procedure is specific for a particular analyte (complete discrimination). In this case a combination of two or more analytical procedures is recommended to achieve the necessary level of discrimination.
- Identification test.
- Presence of closely related structures.
- Confirmed by obtaining positive results from samples containing the analyte, coupled with negative results from samples which do not contain the analyte.
- The choice of such potentially interfering materials should be based on sound scientific judgment with a consideration of the interferences that could occur.

Assay and Impurity Test(s)

- For chromatographic procedures, representative chromatograms should be used to demonstrate specificity.

- Critical separations in chromatography should be investigated for **resolution** at an appropriate level.

- In cases where a non-specific assay is used, other supporting analytical procedures should be used to demonstrate overall specificity.

Resolution in chromatography

- The **resolution** of a elution is a quantitative measure of how well two elution peaks can be differentiated in a **chromatographic** separation.

- It is defined as the difference in retention times between the two peaks, divided by the combined widths of the elution peaks.

- R of > 2 between the peak of interest and the closest potential interfering peak (impurity, excipient, degradation product, internal standard, etc.) is desirable.

$$R = \frac{t_{R2} - t_{R1}}{\frac{1}{2}(W_1 + W_2)} \qquad \ldots\ldots(5.1)$$

$$R = 1.18 \times \left(\frac{t_{R2} - t_{R1}}{(W_{0.5h1} + W_{0.5h2})} \right) \qquad \ldots\ldots(5.2)$$

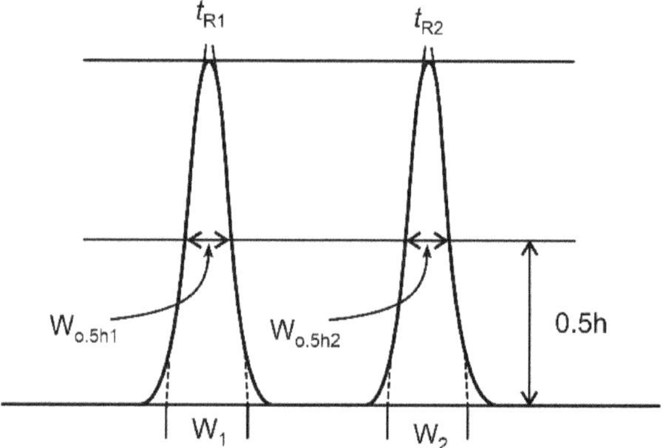

t_{R1}, t_{R2} : Retention time for each peak ($t_{R1} > t_{R2}$)

$W_{0.5h1}, W_{0.5h2}$:Full width at half maximum (FWHM) of each peak

W_1, W_2 :Width of each peak

Figure 5.1 Two Adjacent Peaks.

Assay and Impurity Test(s)

Impurities are available

- For the assay

This should involve demonstration of the discrimination of the analyte in the presence of impurities and/or excipients.

Practically, this can be done by spiking pure substances (drug substance or drug product) with appropriate levels of impurities and/or excipients and demonstrating that the assay result is unaffected by the presence of these materials (by comparison with the assay result obtained on unspiked samples).

Assay and Impurity Test(s)

Impurities are available

The discrimination may be established by spiking drug substance or drug product with appropriate levels of impurities and demonstrating the separation of these impurities individually and/or from other components in the sample matrix.

Impurities are not available

- For the impurity tests, the impurity profiles should be compared.
- Peak purity tests may be useful to show that the analyte chromatographic peak is not attributable to more than one component (e.g., diode array, mass spectrometry).

2. **Linearity**
   - The linearity of an analytical procedure is its ability (within a given range) to obtain test results which are directly proportional to the concentration (amount) of analyte in the sample.
   - For the establishment of linearity, a minimum of 5 concentrations is recommended.
   - Other approaches should be justified.

3. **Range**
   - The range of an analytical procedure is the interval between the upper and lower concentration (amounts) of analyte in the sample (including these concentrations) for which it has been demonstrated that the analytical procedure has a suitable level of precision, accuracy and linearity.
   - The specified range is normally derived from linearity studies and depends on the intended application of the procedure.

The following minimum specified ranges should be considered:

- For the assay of a drug substance or a finished (drug) product: normally from 80 to 120 percent of the test concentration;

- For content uniformity, covering a minimum of 70 to 130 percent of the test concentration, unless a wider more appropriate range, based on the nature of the dosage form, is justified;

- For dissolution testing: +/-20 % over the specified range;

- for the determination of an impurity: from the reporting level of an impurity to 120% of the specification;

- For impurities known to be unusually potent or to produce toxic or unexpected pharmacological effects, the detection/quantitation limit should be commensurate with the level at which the impurities must be controlled.

4. Calibration curve

Definition

It is the relationship between known concentrations and experimental response values (Instrument responses).

Goal

To determine the unknown concentration of a sample

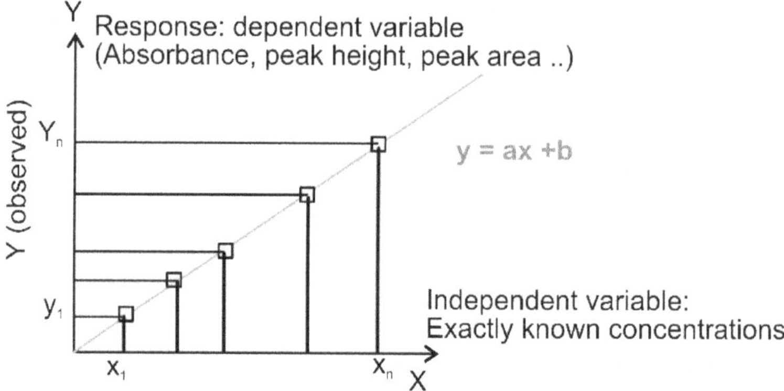

- Construction

5 to 8 points over the analytical domain

replicates are required to test linearity

3 to 5 replicates per levels

The calibration curve should be prepared in the same biological matrix (e.g. plasma) as the sample in the intended study by spiking with known concentration of the analyte (or by serial dilution).

Reference Standard

- Calibration standards and quality control samples (QC)
- Authenticated analytical reference standard should be used to prepare (separately) solution of known concentration
- Certified reference standards
  (Never from a marketed drug formulation)
- Commercially supplied reference standards
- Other material of documented purity

5. Accuracy and precision

Accuracy

The accuracy of an analytical procedure expresses the closeness of agreement between the value which is accepted either as a conventional true value or an accepted reference value and the value found.

Precision

The precision of an analytical procedure expresses the closeness of agreement (degree of scatter) between a series of measurements obtained from multiple sampling of the same homogeneous sample under the prescribed conditions.

Accuracy and precision

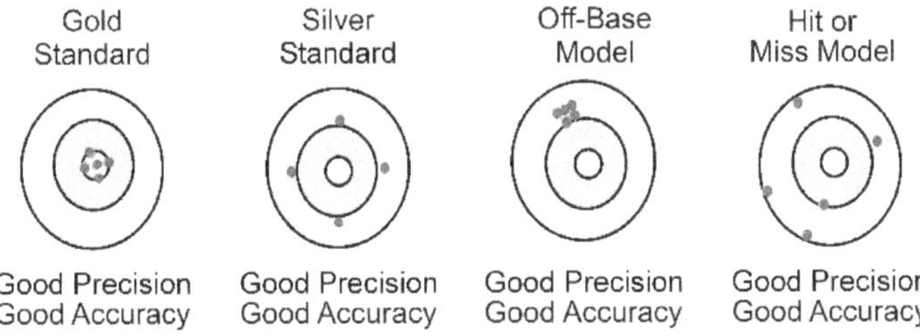

Estimation of Precision

Should be measured using 3 replicates of 3 QC samples

The precision at each concentration should not exceed 15%, except for the LQC (20%)

Within day (Intra-day): Express the precision under the same operating conditions over a short interval of time. Also referred to as Intra-assay precision

Between day (Inter-day)

Intra-day Precision: data analysis

- Precision is calculated on CV% (coefficient of variance)
- Single level of concentration with repetition
  e.g. 12, 13, 12, 14, 13, 14 µg/mL

- mean : 13.0 µg/mL
- SD: 0.8944 µg/mL
- CV% = SD/mean * 100 = 6.88%
- CV% is also known as the relative standard deviation or RSD

Precision may be considered at three levels:

- Repeatability,
- Intermediate precision
- Reproducibility

Repeatability

- Repeatability expresses the precision under the same operating conditions over a short interval of time. Repeatability is also termed intra-assay precision.
- A minimum of 9 determinations covering the specified range for the procedure (e.g., 3 concentrations/3 replicates each).

or

- A minimum of 6 determinations at 100% of the test concentration.

Intermediate precision

- Intermediate precision expresses within-laboratories variations: different days, different analysts, different equipment, etc.

Reproducibility

- Reproducibility expresses the precision between laboratories (collaborative studies, usually applied to standardization of methodology).

Determination of accuracy

$$\text{Accuracy (\%)} = 100 \times \frac{\text{Found value} - \text{Theoretical value}}{\text{Theoritical value}}$$

Determination

- By replicate analysis of the sample containing known amount of analyte
- Minimum 3 replicates of 3 QC samples
- The mean value should be within 15% of the actual value except at LQC where it should not deviate by more than 20%
- Determine intra-day and inter-day accuracy

6. Limit of detection (LOD)

- The detection limit of an individual analytical procedure is the lowest amount of analyte in a sample which can be detected but not necessarily quantitated as an exact value.

- Several approaches for determining the quantitation limit are possible, depending on whether the procedure is a non-instrumental or instrumental. Approaches other than those listed here may be acceptable.

- Based on Visual Evaluation

- Based on Signal to Noise (S/N) ratio of 3:1

- Based on the Standard Deviation of the Response and the Slope

$$DL = \frac{3.3\sigma}{S}$$

where σ = the standard deviation of the response

S = the slope of the calibration curve

- Determination of σ of the response

- Based on Standard Deviation of the Blank

- Based on the Calibration Curve

- The detection limit and the method used for determining the detection limit should be presented. If LOD is determined based on visual evaluation or based on signal to noise ratio, the presentation of the relevant chromatograms is considered acceptable for justification.

7. Limit of quantification (LOQ)

- The quantitation limit of an individual analytical procedure is the lowest amount of analyte in a sample which can be quantitatively determined with suitable precision and accuracy.

- The quantitation limit is a parameter of quantitative assays for low levels of compounds in sample matrices, and is used particularly for the determination of impurities and/or degradation products.

The response (e.g analyte peak) has a precision of 20% and accuracy 80-120%

Based on Visual Evaluation

Based on Signal to Noise (S/N) ratio of 10:1

Based on the Standard Deviation of the Response and the Slope

$$QL = \frac{10\sigma}{S}$$

where σ = the standard deviation of the response

   S = the slope of the calibration curve

- Determination of σ of the response

Based on Standard Deviation of the Blank

Based on the Calibration Curve

- The detection limit and the method used for determining the detection limit should be presented. If LOQ is determined based on visual evaluation or based on signal to noise ratio, the presentation of the relevant chromatograms is considered acceptable for justification.

8. Recovery:

- The recovery of an analyte in an assay is the detector response obtained from an amount of the analyte added to and extracted from the biological matrix, compared to the detector response obtained for the true concentration of the pure authentic standard.

- The recovery allows to determine the percent of lost drug during sample preparation.

- Absolute recovery is evaluated using low, medium, and high QC samples and at least three times for each level.

- The extraction recovery of the analyte (s) and internal standard(s) should be higher than 70%, precise, and reproducible.

9. Ruggedness

Degree of reproducibility of test results under a variety of conditions

(a) Different Laboratories

(b) Different Analysts

(c) Different Instruments

(d) Different Reagents

Expressed as %RSD

10. Robustness

- The robustness of an analytical procedure is a measure of its capacity to remain unaffected by small, but deliberate variations in method parameters and provides an indication of its reliability during normal usage.

- Determination: Comparison of results (precision) under differing conditions to that under normal conditions.

- Examples of typical variations in LC

- (a) Influence of variations of pH in a mobile phase
- (b) Influence of variations in mobile phase composition
- (c) Different columns (different lots and/or suppliers)
- (d) Temperature
- (e) Flow rate

- Examples of typical variations in GC
  - (a) Different columns (different lots and/or suppliers)
  - (b) Temperature
  - (c) Flow rate

- If measurements are susceptible to variations in analytical conditions, the analytical conditions should be suitably controlled or a precautionary statement should be included in the procedure.

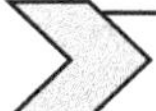

5.3   Calibration

- Calibration of an instrument is the process of determining its accuracy.

- The process involves obtaining a reading from the instrument and measuring its variation from the reading obtained from a standard instrument.

- Calibration of an instrument also involves adjusting its precision and accuracy so that its readings come in accordance with the established standard.

Why calibrate?

There are three main reasons for having instruments calibrated.

- ➢ To ensure readings from an instrument are consistent with other measurements.

- ➢ To determine the accuracy of the instrument readings.

- ➢ To establish the reliability of the instrument i.e. that it can be trusted.

When to calibrate?

- A measuring device should be calibrated.
- According to recommendation of the manufacturer.
- After any mechanical or electrical shock.
- Periodically (annually, quarterly, monthly).
- When a specified usage (operating hours) has elapsed.
- After an instrument has been repaired or modified.
- Whenever observations appear questionable.

- Calibrate too often is waste of time & money.
- Calibrate too seldom is waste of product.
- Sudden changes in weather.
- A new instrument.
- Some experiments required calibration certificates. Check the requirements first before starting the experiment.
- Before major critical measurements.

What is tolerance?

- Tolerance is the greatest range of variation that can be allowed for an instrument or equipment.
- How to determine the tolerance interval?
  - ➢ To determine the tolerance interval in a measurement, add and subtract one-half of the precision of the measuring instrument to the measurement.
  - ➢ For example: if a measurement made with a 10 mL pipette is 5.6 mL and the pipette has a precision of 0.1 mL, then the tolerance interval in this measurement is 5.6 plus minus 0.05 mL, or from 5.55 mL to 5.65 mL.
- Any measurements within this range are "tolerated" or perceived as correct.

5.3.1 Calibration of pH Meter

- pH is defined as the negative decimal logarithm of the hydrogen ion activity.
- pH scale is based on the pH values of a series of standard buffer solutions determined by the potentiometric technique.
- Routine potentiometric measurements of pH are carried out by means of a pH meter equipped by a pH-indicator glass electrode, a reference electrode and an automatic temperature compensator.

5.3.2 How a pH Meter Works

- There are two electrodes in a pH meter, and both are submerged into the solution. One of the electrodes is a glass electrode probe that emits a small voltage and measures the quantity of hydrogen ions attracted to it. The reference probe is electrically neutral. The charge difference between the two probes displays as a pH measurement on the meter.
- pH meters measure the electrical potential produced by a solution and then compare it to known solutions. Calibration of a pH meter is done

using measuring substances with known pH levels, called buffers, and setting the pH measurements to those levels on the pH meter.

- The pH meter uses the calibration measurements as a guide in the measuring of other substances. pH meters lose some of their accuracy with every use, and the calibration of a pH meter must be completed often if not daily.

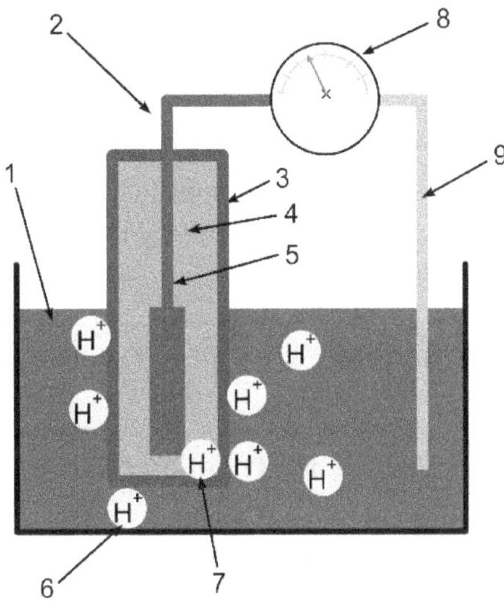

1) Solution being tested; (2) Glass electrode, consisting of (3) a thin layer of silica glass containing metal salts, inside which there is a potassium chloride solution (4) and an internal electrode (5) made from silver/silver chloride. (6) Hydrogen ions formed in the test solution interact with the outer surface of the glass. (7) Hydrogen ions formed in the potassium chloride solution interact with the inside surface of the glass. (8) The meter measures the difference in voltage between the two sides of the glass and converts this "potential difference" into a pH reading. (9) Reference electrode acts as a baseline or reference for the measurement—or you can think of it as simply completing the circuit.

5.3.3 Procedure

Use the following four steps in the calibration of pH meters.

Step 1: Clean the Electrodes

- If working with laboratory equipment and chemicals, it is important to wear proper safety equipment, such as gloves and safety glasses. After turning on the power to the pH meter, take the pH meter electrode from its storage solution and rinse with distilled water. Wipe it clean with a lint-free tissue.

Step 2: Calibrate With the pH 7 Buffer

- Submerge the rinsed electrode into the pH 7 buffer solution. Press the calibrate button and wait for the pH icon to stop flashing. If the pH reads 7, accept; if it does not, edit the entry using the keypad on the instrument. Rinse the electrode again with distilled water and wipe clean with a lint-free tissue.

Step 3: Calibrate With the pH 10 and 4 Buffer

- Now submerge the rinsed electrode into the pH 10 buffer. Press the calibrate button once the pH icon stops flashing. If the pH reads 10, accept; if it does not, edit the entry using the keypad on the instrument. Rinse the electrode with distilled water and wipe with a lint-free tissue. Repeat the same for pH 4 buffer.

Step 4: Measure the pH of Solutions

- The pH meter is now ready to measure the pH of other substances. Be sure to submerge the electrode and rinse with distilled water in between multiple samples.

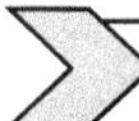

5.4   Qualification

- The validation of a process requires the qualification of each of the important elements of the process.
- The relative importance of an element may vary from process to process. the elements commonly considered in a process validation study are:
- Design qualification
- Installation qualification
- Operational qualification
- Performance qualification

Scope

Documented evidence to prove that:

- Premises
- Supporting utilities
- Equipment

have been **designed** in accordance with GMP

- Also referred as **Design Qualification (DQ)** where appropriate.

5.4.1   Design Qualification

- The first element of validation of new facilities, systems or equipment could be design qualification (DQ).
- The compliance of the design with GMP should be demonstrated and documented.

Scope

Documented evidence to prove that:

- Premises
- Supporting utilities
- Equipment

have been built and installed in accordance with their design specifications.

5.4.2   Installation Qualification

- IQ is a method of establishing with confidence that all major processing, packaging equipment and ancillary systems are in conformance with installation specifications, equipment manuals, schematics and engineering drawings.
- This stage of validation includes examination of equipment design, determination of calibration, maintenance and adjustment requirements.

IQ must include

- Installation of equipment, piping, services and instrumentation checked to current engineering drawings and specifications.
- Collection and collation of supplier operating and working instructions and maintenance requirements.
- Calibration requirements.
- Verification of materials of construction.
- Description of equipment.
- Piping and Instrument diagrams.
- Principle of operation.
- Facility functional specifications.
- Design requirements.
- Equipment utility requirements, equipment specification, equipment features.

Scope

Documented evidence to prove that:

- Supporting utilities
- Equipment

operate in accordance with their design specifications.

5.4.3   Operational Qualification

- The conduct of an operational qualification (OQ) should follow an authorized protocol.

- The critical operating parameters for the equipment and systems should be identified at the OQ stage.

- The plans for the OQ should identify the studies to be undertaken on the critical variables, the sequence of those studies and the measuring equipment to be used and the acceptance criteria to be met.

- Studies on the critical variables should include a condition or a set of conditions encompassing upper and lower processing and operating limits referred to as "worst-case" conditions.

- The completion of a successful OQ should allow the finalization of operating procedures and operator instructions documentation for the equipment.

- This information should be used as the basis for training of operators in the requirements for satisfactory operation of the equipment.

OQ should include

- Tests that have been developed from knowledge of processes, systems and equipment.

- Tests to include a condition or a set of conditions encompassing upper and lower operating limits, sometimes referred to as "worst case" conditions.

- The completion of a successful Operational qualification should allow the finalization of calibration, operating and cleaning procedures, operator training and preventive maintenance requirements. It should permit a formal "release" of the facilities, systems and equipment.

- Equipment operational procedures established and challenged.

- Equipment control functions.

- Calibration requirements & schedules established.

- Maintenance requirements & established schedules.

Scope

Documented evidence to prove that, e.g.

- Supporting utilities
- Equipment

perform consistently in accordance with their design specifications.

5.4.4   Performance Qualification

Performance qualification (PQ) should follow successful completion of Installation qualification and Operational qualification. PQ should include, but not be limited to the following:

- Tests, using production materials, qualified substitutes or simulated product, that have been developed from knowledge of the process and the facilities, systems or equipment.

- Tests to include a condition or set of conditions encompassing upper and lower operating limits.

- Although PQ is described as a separate activity, it may in some cases be appropriate to perform it in conjunction with OQ. Qualification of established (in-use) facilities, systems and equipment.

- Additionally, the calibration, cleaning, preventive maintenance, operating procedures and operator training procedures and records should be documented.

Scope

- Documented evidence to prove that:

A specific process will consistently produce a product meeting its predetermined specifications and quality attributes

- Also referred to as Process Validation (PV)

What should be qualified?

Applicable to any aspect of operation which may affect the quality of the product:

- Directly or indirectly.

- Cover e.g. premises, facilities (utilities), equipment, processes.

- In case of significant changes – consider the need for re-qualification or re-validation.

Principle

- Qualification and validation should be done in accordance with an ongoing program:

- Initial qualification and validation

- Annual review (determine the need for re-validation)

- Ensure continued validation status is maintained.

- Policy described in relevant documentation, e.g. quality manual, or Validation Master Plan (VMP).

Operational qualification and performance verification of UV-visible spectrophotometers

Design Qualification (DQ)

- DQ provides an opportunity for the user to demonstrate that the instrument's fitness for purpose

- Establish the intended or likely use of the instrument and should define an appropriate user requirement specification (URS)

Fully documented quality control and quality assurance procedures, including

- Design and specification;

- Suitably qualified and experienced personnel;

- Comprehensive and planned testing of all parts of the system, and;

- Stringent change control, error reporting and corrective procedures.

Design qualification - general considerations

Feature	Consideration
Instrument set-up & Control	PC based or integrated system. Software control of operating conditions and parameters. Data acquisition, processing and presentation needs. In-built diagnostic facilities. Self-testing diagnostics. Detector options. Source options.
Sample introduction & Throughput	Sample throughput, presentation and introduction needs. Sample thermostatting requirements. Sample volume requirements.
Materials of Construction	Resistance to corrosion, contamination by solvents and samples.
Installation Requirements	Size and weight in shipped form. Access restrictions to permanent site.
Operational Requirements	Limitations on, requirements for and expected consumption of services, utilities, and consumables (e.g. lamps). Ventilation requirements. Controlling sofware embedded or separate package.

Design qualification of UV-Vis instruments

Feature	Consideration
System control and communication*	Spectrometer parameters selected/controlled/stored/retrieved either locally within the optical instrument, or via a remote PC or system controller. Ability to send/accept/store/retrieve signals (e.g. through contact closures) and to communicate (e.g. RS232) with other devices.

Table *contd...*

Feature	Consideration
Source type	Lamp life, warm-up time, susceptibility to drigt. Wavelength at which lamp changes (if at all).
Samples*	Sample types accommodated (conventional, turbid, solid). Ability to handle discrete samples (single cell or matched cells) or continuous (flowcell). Range of sample sizes possible (cell volume and path length, minimum flushing volume for floecells) Ability to handle multiple samples either attended or unattended, and possible match size. Facility for control sample cell temperature: range (including sub-ambient facility), accuracy, stability, type (Peltier or circulating). Ease of interchange of different cell types or accessories
Detector type	Ability to monitor single, multiple or variable wavelengths and/or full spectral characteristics, required acquisition speed of full spectra.
Wavelength accuracy	Ability to select required wavelengths accurately and reproducibly.
Wavelength range	Ability to select and monitor required wavelengths, with or without changing source, filter or detector.
Linear dynamic range	Ability for accurate quantitation over a large absorbance range.
Optical and electronic noise	Low noise facilitates improved sensitivity and lower detection limits (note whether peak-to peak or RMS).
Wavelength drift	Low drift facilitates improved sensitivity and lower detection limits.
Resolution	Important for accurate measurement of narrow bands.
Photometric accuracy	Good accuracy required for absolute absorbance measurements.

Installation qualification (IQ)

- Has the instrument been delivered as ordered, e.g. according to the DQ or purchase order?

- Has the instrument been checked and verified as undamaged?

- Has the appropriate documentation been supplied, is it of correct issue and uniquely identified by part number, version number and date?

- Have details of all services and utilities required to operate the instrument been provided (preferably in advance of the delivery)?

- Is it clear which maintenance, calibration and performance tests should be carried out by the user and which by the supplier or their agent.

- Have details of recommended service and calibration intervals (carried out by the supplier) been provided?

- Have intervals, methods and instructions for user-maintenance and calibration been provided along with contact points for service and spare parts?

- Has the correct hardware, firmware and software been supplied and is it of correct issue and uniquely identified by part number?

- Has information been provided on consumables required during the normal operation of the instrument system?

- Is the selected environment for the instrument system suitable, with adequate room for packing, installation, operation and servicing, and have appropriate services and utilities (electricity, water, etc.) been provided?

- Has health and safety and environmental information relating to the operation of the instrument been provided and is the proposed working environment consistent with these requirements?

- Is the response of the instrument to the initial application of power as expected and have any deviations been recorded?

Performance qualification

Performance Tests	Standards	Pharmacopoeia[a]			
		USP 26	BP 2001	EP 4 Ed.	JP (XIV)
Wavelength accuracy	Deuterium lamp	√	√	√	√
	Mercury vapor lamp	√	√	√	√
	Holmium oxide glass filter	√			√
	Didymium glass filter	√			√
	Holmium oxide in HClO4	√	√	√	
Wavelength reproducibility					√
Stray light	Potassium chloride solution (200 nm)		√	√	
	Potassium iodide solution (220 nm)	√			
Resolution	Toluene in hexane solution		√	√	
Photometric accuracy	Neutral-density glass filters	√			
	Mental on quartz filters	√			
	Potassium dichromate solution	√	√	√	√
Photometric reproducibility	Potassium dichromate solution				
Noise					
Baseline flatness					
Stability					
Linearity					

5.4.5 Performance Tests for UV-Vis Spectrophotometers

- Performance attributes
- Wavelength Accuracy

Wavelength accuracy is defined as the deviation of the wavelength reading at an absorption band or emission band from the known wavelength of the band.

Holmium oxide solution is commercially available in a sealed 1-cm cuvette.

It is a very convenient and versatile wavelength standard

Acceptance: ± 1 nm in the UV range (200 to 380 nm) and ± 3 nm in the visible range (380 to 800 nm). Three repeated scans of the same peak should be within ±0.5 nm

Effect of wavelength accuracy on UV–Vis measurements

- Holmium oxide solution available in a sealed 1-cm cuvette.
- It is a very convenient and versatile wavelength standard.
- Spectral bandwidth ranging from 2 to 0.5 nm.

Acceptance. ± 1 nm in the UV range (200 to 380 nm) and ± 3 nm in the visible range (380 to 800 nm). Three repeated scans of the same peak should be within ±0.5 nm.

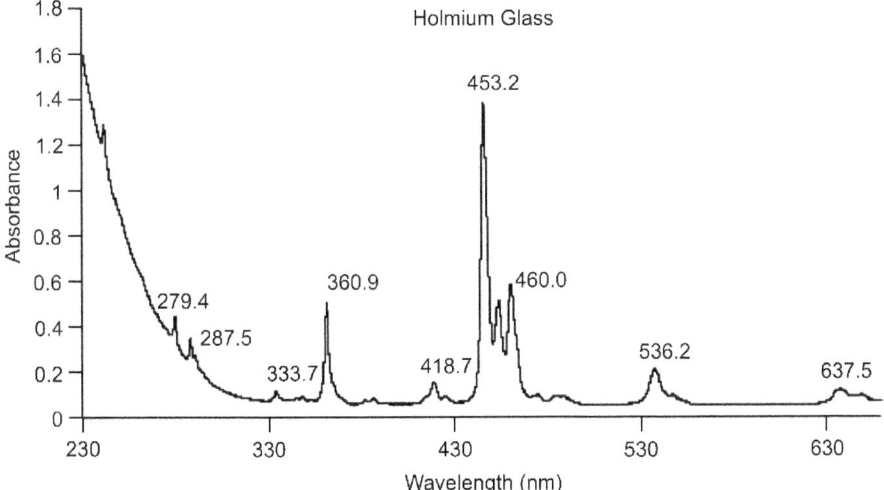

Absorption spectrum of holmium oxide filter

Wavelength standard comparison

Wavelength standard	Advantages	Disadvantages
Emission lines from deuterium lamp	Sharp spectral lines Present in the UV light source	Limited to visible wavelengths (486.0 and 656.1 nm)
Emission lines from mercury vapor lamp	Sharp spectral lines Covers both UV and visible regions	Not commonly built into the instrument
Holmium oxide and didymium filters	Easy to use NIST SRM available	Glass filter absorbs strongly below 300 nm: limited to mainly visible wavelengths (280-640 nm) Broad spectral lines Recertification required every two years
4% Holmium oxide in 10% perchloric acid	Easy to use NIST SRM available (2034) Covers both UV and visible regions (240-650 nm) Recertification required every eight years	Dependency on the resolution of the instrument Corrosive solution

Stray light

High-absorbance measurements are affected more severely by stray light.

$$\text{Absorbance (A)} = -\log \text{transmittance (T)}$$

where T is the ratio of intensity of the transmitted light (I) and incident light (I 0). In the presence of stray light,

$$T = \frac{I + I_s}{I_0 + I_s}$$

where *Is* is intensity of the stray light. If there is no stray light, the absorbance value should be 2.

I_s (Stray Light)	I_i (Transmitted)	$I = I_s + I_i$	I_o	$T = I / I_o$	$A = -\log T$
0%	1%	1%	100.0%	0.0100	2.000
0.1%	1%	1.01%	100.1%	0.0101	1.996
0.5%	1%	1.05%	100.5%	0.0149	1.826
1%	1%	2%	101.0%	0.0198	1.703

Resolution

Insufficient resolution leads to a decrease in the extinction coefficient across the wavelength axis, and therefore inaccurate quantitation results.

A solution mixture of 0.02% v/v toluene in hexane (UV grade) is used to test the resolution power of the spectrophotometer.

Acceptance. The ratio of the absorbance at λ_{max} (269 nm) and absorbance at λ_{min} (266 nm) should be greater than 1.5.

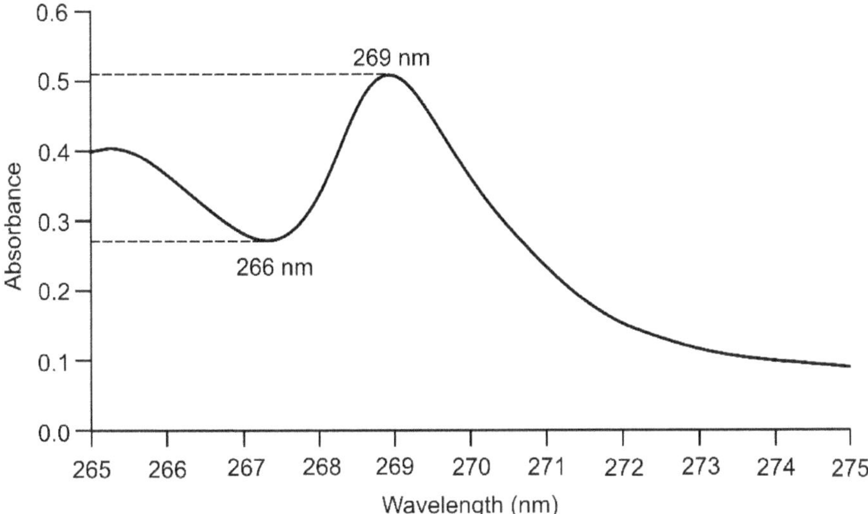

Noise

Noise in the UV–Vis measurement originates primarily from the light source and electronic components.

Tests. Air is scanned in the absorbance mode for 10 min. peak-to-peak noise is recorded at 500 nm. The root mean square (RMS) noise is calculated.

Acceptance. The RMS noise should typically be less than 0.001 AU.

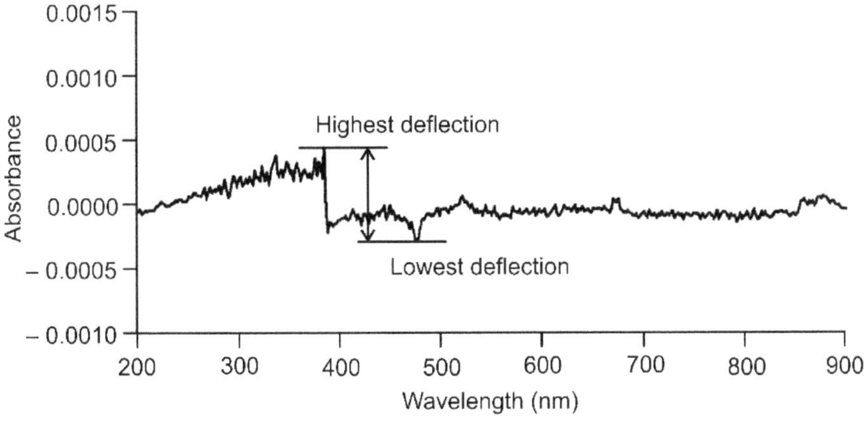

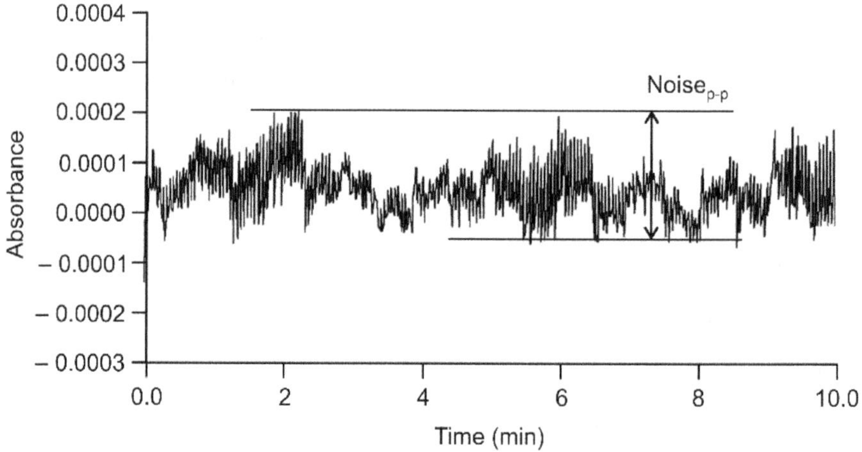

5.5   Good Warehousing Practice

Introduction: Maintaining proper storage condition for pharmaceutical products and paramedical is vital to ensure their quality, safety and efficacy. Factory stores will invariably be receiving duly approved raw materials and packaging materials from third party. A suitable space is provided to raw material, handling of raw & packaging materials required for manufacturing, including packaging of pharmaceuticals. This space is known as Warehouse. It is a part of pharmaceutical company.

For what purpose? To enable the fastest and cheapest transport of drugs and medical equipment from suppliers to beneficiaries. There are mainly 3 stages:

1. Purchase of pharmaceutical products.
2. Storage of ordered products.
3. Distribution of stocked products.

5.5.1   Various Areas of Warehousing

- **RECEIVING AREA:** includes initial inspection, cleaning & weight checking.

- **SAMPLING AREA:** with adequate facilities to prevent cross contamination.

- **STORAGE AREA:** including specific storage like air

- **STORAGE AREA:** including specific storage like air condition rooms, cold rooms, hazardous chemical storage room.

- **DISPENSING AREA:** with adequate facilities to preclude cross contamination during dispensing.

Design

Principle: Premises must be located, designed, constructed, adapted, and maintained to suit the operations to be carried out.

General

- The layout and design of premises must aim to minimize the risk of errors and permit effective cleaning and maintenance in order to avoid cross-contamination, build-up of dust or dirt, and, in general, any adverse effect on the quality of products.

- Where dust is generated (e.g. during sampling, weighing, mixing and processing operations, packaging of powder), measures should be taken to avoid cross-contamination and facilitate cleaning.

- Premises should be situated in an environment in which the minimum risk of any contamination of materials or products.

- Premises used for the manufacture of finished products should be suitably designed and constructed to facilitate good sanitation.

- Premises should be carefully maintained, and it should be ensured that repair and maintenance operations do not causes any hazard to the quality of products.

- Premises should be cleaned and, where applicable, disinfected according to detailed written procedures. Records should be maintained.

- Electrical supply, lighting, temperature, humidity and ventilation should be appropriate and such that they do not adversely affect, directly or indirectly, either the pharmaceutical products during their manufacture and storage, or the accurate functioning of equipment.

- Premises should be designed and equipped so as to afford maximum protection against the entry of insects, birds or other animals. There should be a standard procedure to prevent from rodent and pest control.

- Premises should be designed to ensure the logical flow of materials and personnel.

5.5.2 Good Warehousing Practice

- Factory Stock which should be received with proper documents detailing the names of product, the batch number, the number of units of final packs of each batch, the date of   dispatch and the quality control status of the batches.

- The stock control system must be such that only passed batches of products are issued for distribution. Stocks should be stored, product wise to enable quick identification and control of stock movement.

- Stocks should therefore be racked and stored in a manner that earlier stocks are earlier accessible than the later ones.

- The picking and assembling areas should be so arranged as to minimize the distance travelled by warehouse operators. Picking stocks should be located on shelves at convenient heights and with proper labels which clearly identify the products.

- Assembled products should be checked for accuracy of quantities and identities of products ordered. Batch details should be recorded in relevant documents.

- Finished product should be packed in the containers and dispatched for the transportation.

- The unit product packs should be not contaminated by other products. Vehicles which carry the final packaged stocks of products should be so selected that-

  1. They are clear, dry and sufficiently protected from rain and other weather factors.

  2. They are free from infestation.

  3. They do not give off strong odours which may contaminate the products.

  4. They are suitable to withstand the weight of the load they carry.

5.5.3   Storage of Raw & Packaging Materials

Storage Condition- special storage area with controlled temperature, humidity & stored off from the floor.

Storage of Packaging Material
- Bottles, vials, ampoules, tins, tubes should be stored in a manner that they do not contaminated by extraneous matter.

- Printed packaging material also stored properly.

- Printed materials such as labels, printed films / foils /laminates, cartons should keep in storage cupboards.

- Preventing mix up of printed & non printed materials.

- Physical segregation of printed & labeled containers should be made.

- Special precautions are needed for the storage of —packaging labeling controlled products.

- Appropriate storage condition to be provided (air conditioning, aluminum foil)

5.5.4 Handling & Issue – Raw Materials

- Attention to be made for   -prevent cross contamination, health of personnel handling materials, containers should be closed properly, materials that support microbial growth are handled carefully. Eg. agar.
- Materials issued only against authorized person.
- Personnel protective devices like gloves, facemasks etc. should be used to avoid health hazards. Adequate dust extraction system should be provided to suck away fine dust as to prevent cross-contamination.

5.5.5 Handling & Issue: Packaging Materials

- Packaging materials issued to production only against packaging materials order.
- Care should made to check for only right packaging materials to be issued.
- Unlike raw materials, exact quantity of packaging materials to be issued.
- Unused packaging materials returned to the warehouse & will accompanied by authorized documents
- For avoiding deterioration, spoilage or breakage

Requirements

Safe, orderly & dispatch of all products -cold storage area have temperature monitoring & recording devices -racking & shelving system should have good mechanical strength.

Procedure: Stock received from factory with proper documentation (name, batch number, date of dispatch)

Finished products which are —under test" must be quarantined & segregated from —passed stocks"

Stock should be stored product wise to enable quick identification & controlled stock movement

Store rotation should be on —first in, first out basis.

5.5.6 Stock Management

Objectives

- To ensure continuity of supplies.
- To avoid over stocking.

Stock management will set out to;

- monitor stock levels

- monitor consumption

- anticipate delivery time for order activation.

Issuing of material

- store should issue raw and packaging materials on the basis of FIFO (first come first out) basis. Entry and exit of every consignment of materials should be entered on the stock card.

- Issuing of materials should do on the basis of raw and packaging materials required in manufacturing process. while issuing hazardous and explosive materials, the operation should be supervised to prevent any mistake.

5.5.7   Material Management

1. **Intermediate:** In Pharmaceutical industry normally main or central warehouse is responsible for the management of raw material, Packaging and Finished Products. However, intermediate and bulk product storage is responsibility of the production department.

   Intermediate/ Bulk Product may be defined as the material which has started processing but not yet converted into finished products.

   - Granulated material for compression.

   - Compressed tablet for coating and Packaging.

   - Filter and Un-filtered liquid for oral and injectable.

   These Products should be kept under appropriate storage condition of temperature, R.H (Relative humidity), Clean of air etc.

2. **Reagents and Culture Media:**   The following points should be considered regarding management of reagents and culture media:

   (i)   All reagents and cultures media should be recorded on Receipt and Prepn.

   (ii) Reagents made up in the laboratories should be prepared according to the written procedure and appropriate labelled such labelled should indicate following information:

   a. Name of the Reagent.

   b. Nominal conc.

   c. Shelf life.

   d. Standardization vector.

   e. Date when Standardization is required.

   f. Storage Condition.

   g. Name, Signature and date of Person who has prepared and Standardized the Reagents.

(iii) A registered should be Maintained giving detail of reagents maintained standardized, re-standardized, used in destroyed if any.

(iv) Both positive and negative controls should be applied to verified suitability of culture media.

3. **Waste Materials:** Pharmaceutical Manufacturing operations generate lots of waste materials. These materials can be classified into 2 categories:

   a. Trash

   b. Scarp

(i) **Trash:** Which don't have any resale value and may be disposed by proper method depending on the nature of the trash.

(ii) **Scarp:** Which don't have resale value and may be sold to scarp dealers after proper Segregation.

- Provisions Should be made for proper and safe storage of waste materials. Toxic substances and flammable materials should be stored in suitability enclosed cupboards.

- Before disposal of these materials, they can be separated in diff. categories: - Paper, Aluminum foil, Metal Containers, Plastic, Glan.

- Safety of Materials to be disposed must be considered.

4. **Reference Standards:** May be available in the form of official reference standard.

- Reference standards by producers should be tested released than stored in the same way as official standards.

- They should be kept under responsibility for designated person in a secure area.

- Official reference standard should be used only for the purposed described in the appropriate monograph.

- Secondary or working standard may be established by the application of appropriate test and checks at regular intervals to ensure standardization.

- All such reference standard should be stored and used in manner that will not adversely affect their quality.

   1. **Packaging Material**

      (i) **Primary Packaging Materials:** Materials which come in contact directly with the medicinal product. e.g. Bottle and Tubes.

    (ii) Secondary Packaging Materials: Materials which come in contact with the primary materials.

    (iii) Printed Packaging Materials: All packaging material which have anything printed on it such materials include label on it. It includes cartoon, foils etc.

    (iv) Tertiary and other Packaging materials: All Packaging materials other than those covered in these 3 known as $3^{®}$ Packaging materials.

5.5.8 Handling of these Materials

- These purchase handling and control of primary and printed packaging material shall be as for Raw Material.

- Printed Packaging material should be stored securely lock and key system to avoid un-authorized access.

- A detailed SOP's should be available for dispensing of PM's. only authorized personnel should do dispensing and make records of all the activities.

- Each delivery or batch of printed or primary PM's should be given a specific reference number or identification marks.

- Outdated and absolute primary PM should be destroyed by suitable and approved method of distribution and records are maintained.

- The destruction of PPM's should be done under the supervision of a responsible and QA Person.

- All Product and PM to be should be checked and delivered to the packaging department for quality, identity and conformity.

- Accesses to all storage areas should be limited to the authorized persons only.

- A separate sampling room should be provided for sampling of PPM which should be fairly cleaned.

  1. **Finished Products:** These are the products which are in marketable pack. These Product should be held in quarantine until their final release after which they should be stored as un usable stock under conditions established by manufacturer.

     - Each batch of the finished product should be treated as per lay down testing procedure against its specification and then only released for only distributed on or sale.

     - Products failing to meet the established specification or any other relevant quality criteria should be rejected. Reprocessing may be performed if feasible but the reprocess product should meet all the specifications and other quality criteria prior to its.

2. **Recovered and Rejected Products:** Rejected material may be defined as material at any stage which have been tested against a set of predefined specifications and found not to meet the specifications fully, we can deal with such materials mainly in 2 ways:

   - **Re-Process and Re-Test:** The Material to see whether it means a specific requirement.

   - **Destroy:** Send it to supplier.

   The following points should be considered in this regard:

   A. **Rejected Material and Product:** It should clearly mark as such and stored separately in restricted area. Such area in industry is normally be painted red in colour to make it distinguishable easily.

   B. **Rejected Production Batches:** Should be in exponential situation. Such re-process should be permitted only if the re-processed batches is going to meet the same specification after reprocessing.

   A detailed record of such reprocess should be given a new number by means of which such batches can be identified as reprocessed batches.

   C. In Addition of all parts of earlier batches confirming to the required quantity into a batch of the same product at predefined stage of manufacturer should be authorized beforehand.

   a. Need for additional testing of any finished products that has been added should be considered by the department.

3. **Returned Goods:** Pharmaceutical product may be return from market for various reasons like quality problem, accidental damage of goods etc. such products when returned from the market have the following actions taken immediately to it:

   (i) Physical examined condition of the goods return also check all the relevant documents. Ask QC department to evaluate the quality of goods received and take a decision an weather this products can be reprocessed and recovered or needs to be destroyed.

   (ii) If it is possible to re processed or recovered than such products after retesting and reprocessing may be considered for relabeling, repackaging and reselling of the same.

   (iii) QC department should evaluate all aspects like condition of received material, time it was first processed etc. along with chemical, microbiological or any other technical evaluation.

(iv) Where even a slightest doubt arises about the quality of the product it should not be considered suitable for reuse and reissued although the basic chemical reprocessing recovered active ingredient may possible.

Any action should be taken recorded.

4. **Recalled Products:** Products which are already distributed or sold may be required at times to be recalled from market for various reason like Substandard quality detected after the product was distributed, damage of goods during transit such recalled products should be clearly identified or restored separately in a separate area until a decision should be take on their fate such decision should be made possible.

5. **Miscellaneous Materials:** All those materials which don't specifically fold under the category of low material or production material, intermediates, bulk and finished pharmaceuticals will be considered under the category of misc. materials. Such materials like insecticide, fumigating agent, sanitizing agent call under this category. These materials should not be permitted to contamination equipment, packaging material or finished products.

www.ingramcontent.com/pod-product-compliance
Lightning Source LLC
LaVergne TN
LVHW021656160726
843514LV00001B/179